WHAT'S UP, DOC?

Understanding Your Common Symptoms

Dr Tom Stuttaford

To my patients

This edition published in the United Kingdom in 2007 by
Little Books Ltd, 48 Catherine Place, London SW1E 6HL.

10 9 8 7 6 5 4 3 2 1

Text copyright © 2007 by Tom Stuttaford
Design and layout copyright © by 2007 Little Books Ltd

A CIP catalogue record for this book is available from the British Library.

ISBN: 978 1 904435 29 7

The author and publisher will be grateful for any information that will
assist them in keeping future editions up-to-date. Although all reasonable care
has been taken in the preparation of this book, neither the publisher, editors nor
the author can accept any liability for any consequences arising from the use
thereof, or the information contained therein.

Printed and bound by Bookmarque Ltd, Croydon

Contents

Introduction

A persistent cough that hasn't cleared up after having the flu more than a month ago? Increasingly breathless? Just two of the many symptoms that should persuade you to visit your doctor at once.

The tragedy is that many of the patients who came to see me for consultations over the years had symptoms of potentially life-threatening conditions for months – even, in some cases, for over a year.

The reasons for these delays varied. Some patients said that they didn't realize the significance of their symptoms, although these warning signals would have rung alarm bells in every doctor. Many said they thought it would be all right to wait another month or two until they were next in London, or until it was time for their next medical check-up.

Others delayed taking action because they didn't want to make a fuss, and feared that if the symptoms later turned out to be innocent, they would have wasted the doctor's time. Not so. There are many simple explanations and benign causes for what could be a potentially dangerous symptom. Yet when a doctor's only role is to offer much-needed reassurance or to treat a relatively unimportant condition, then he or she is delighted.

British medicine would be as successful as that of other western countries if only the general public were more aware of early symptoms that signal possible danger ahead. The earlier a serious condition is diagnosed, the better the chance of a successful cure.

This is, by design, a small pocket book. Only some of the important symptoms which we, doctors and patients, should be looking out for can be mentioned. There are many others. Yet if, as a result of reading this book, one reader finds a symptom that needs urgent treatment and a life is thereby saved, it will have been well worth publishing.

LOOK OUT FOR

Early Signs of Skin Cancer

moles which are growing

changing colour

are of irregular shape

are of an uneven colour

itch, bleed, are scaly or painful

any irregular, inexplicable lump
or scaly thick patch which

bleeds

ulcerates

refuses to heal

1

SURFACE PROBLEMS
Skin and Mouth Diseases

Skin malignancies

Harriet Johnston is a red-headed, pale-skinned Scot who spends her holidays baking in the Mediterranean sun. She doesn't tan easily, but burns. One winter she noticed a large mole on her forearm. It was raised, irregularly shaped with an uneven, notched border, and the colours weren't uniform, but a mixture of mid- and dark-brown and one black patch. 'Doctor,' she asked, 'could this mole be cancerous?'

The doctor said it could, and needed a biopsy. Distinguishing benign from malignant moles is a job that can even tax an expert, but there are a few danger signs that should be watched out for. Any change in a mole or wart, whether size, colour, shape, or thickness, can be significant. If the mole starts to itch, bleed, become scaly or painful, it needs investigating, but these signs or symptoms are frequently not present in the early stages of cancer. If a significantly sized mole suddenly appears, it should be shown to a doctor. Because of her fair complexion and red hair, Harriet kept a careful eye on her skin.

Malignant moles (melanoma) are much more dangerous on the back than on the limbs or chest, where they are not easily visible. Among the danger signs of a malignant mole are an irregular shape: one half doesn't look like the other. The border of the mole also lacks the well-defined, smooth outline of a benign mole, and instead shows notches and irregularities. Also, most malignant moles may be of many different colours: brown in varying shades, even with traces of pink, blue and, of course, black. Some malignant moles are skin-coloured. If the general thickness and any bumps in a mole suddenly increase, it can be a danger sign.

Malignant moles soon become larger than normal moles; most are more than a quarter of an inch across. Large (over three-eighths of an inch), previously benign moles occasionally turn malignant, and these need expert evaluation.

Harriet's mole was removed. She has had no further trouble.

Sores in the mouth

Forty-year-old TV cameraman Gavin Robinson has an exciting life. He rarely visits a dentist, is a heavy smoker, drinks more than he should and often relaxes with a spliff. He found a sore under the back of his tongue, but took little interest in it until he developed an earache. His doctor found the sore. Could it be cancer?

Yes. Any sore, ulcer or unexplained lump on the mouth, lip, gums or tongue that lasts more than a fortnight should be shown to a doctor or dentist. Cases of mouth cancer are increasing. While partially unexplained, it is known to be associated with smoking – particularly if the smoker also drinks to excess or smokes cannabis. By not going to the dentist, the diagnosis in Gavin's case was delayed. Many cases are only detected when they cause earache.

Other causes of sores, ulcers and lumps in the mouth must be considered, including aphthous ulcers (mouth ulcers) – painful sores that usually last for ten days; cold sores (herpes simplex); thrush, particularly on the tongue or the angles of the mouth; and traumatic sores and ulcers from ill-fitting dentures, sharp teeth, etc.

Potentially malignant rashes and sores include leucoplakia: white or grey patches in the mouth, which may be roughened and thick. They can be caused by irritation, and are usually painless. Sometimes they are pre-cancerous, so any firm, thickened patch that doesn't go within two weeks should be shown to a doctor.

Mouth and lip tumours can be benign, but any ulcer, white patch (possibly with red areas) or lump in the mouth, lips or tongue that doesn't heal and disappear within fourteen days should be examined. Any ulcer forming on a previously smooth polyp or lump needs immediate attention. A persistently enlarged lymph gland in the neck or swelling of the salivary glands in front of the ear or under the jaw need investigation. Earache may result from pressure from a gland that has become swollen from cancer that has spread from the mouth.

LOOK OUT FOR

Early Signs of a Heart Attack

sudden onset of pain

central chest pain – often right across the chest

heavy, crushing and constricting chest pain

may go down the left arm and into the thumb

may go up into the jaw and/or neck

associated with sweating

a pale, damp complexion (sometimes with
blueness of the nose, lips, fingers)

Don't Miss

one-fifth of heart attacks which are silent or near silent
patients may misdiagnose them as indigestion or flu

watch out for a breathlessness, swollen ankles and
feet, unusual fatigue and loss of stamina, as when
climbing stairs, running for the bus

occasionally an irregular pulse (fibrillation)

2
DICKY TICKERS
Heart Disease

CHEST PAIN

Peter was fifty-five, stockily built, competitive and ambitious but without any obvious ability. He was a natural worrier, obsessional, often depressed and dominated by his wife and mother. After exercise, he suffered from chest pain, which spread down his left arm. He asked, 'How do I know if the pain in my chest is coming from my heart?'

Although it turned out that Peter had angina, the overwhelming majority of patients who ask their doctor about chest pain don't have heart disease. A study that was carried out several years ago among middle-aged men showed that the most common cause of chest pain in this group stemmed from musculo-skeletal problems such as strained joints and muscles and pressure on nerve roots – *not* heart disease.

Two other problems are frequently confused with the pain of heart disease. Probably the most common is indigestion, particularly when the stomach contents are irritating and inflaming the bottom of the gullet, a condition known as oesophagitis. 'Over-breathing', or hyperventilation, as the result of anxiety and tension may also cause chest pain that is often confused with heart disease.

Peter's doctor would have questioned him carefully about the nature of his chest pain. Although in Peter's case its anginal cause was obvious, if a diagnosis of heart disease is missed, it can have tragic results in many cases. A number of patients who collapse from a coronary thrombosis (see page 18) do so while clasping an indigestion tablet, having failed to recognize the true cause of the previous chest pain.

Whether it is due to angina or as a result of a coronary thrombosis (also known as a myocardial infarction), the pain of coronary heart disease is a gripping pain. Patients describe it as feeling like a steel band being tightened across their chests, or as a heavy feeling, like having a sack of potatoes pressing on the chest. It is usually felt maximally over the centre of the chest, but often extends right across it and, as in Peter's case, down the inside of either arm, but much more often down the left than the right.

The pain may extend up into the throat and neck, even as far as the jaw, when it can be confused with toothache. Sometimes the pain is also felt in the back, nose or the base of the thumb. Real confusion may arise if, as rarely happens, the pain is felt only in the jaw, thumb or tooth. For example, most doctors have had patients who have had teeth removed in a fruitless attempt to cure what was in fact angina.

If the chest pain is caused by a coronary thrombosis – a heart attack following a blocked artery – rather than angina, which is caused by a narrowed artery, the pain is frequently associated with clinical shock: sweating, a grey complexion, collapse, and nausea and vomiting. Simple angina doesn't last more than four hours. It is induced by exercise and usually goes away as soon as the person stops exercising.

Angina pain isn't sharp or stabbing, but crushing and constricting. It doesn't last for days, even for more than an hour or two, unless there has been a coronary thrombosis.

Unlike indigestion, heart pain doesn't vary with the position of the sufferer. It is not helped by either indigestion medication, or by pills or sprays designed to relieve heart pain. Heart pain, when it is caused by angina, is brought on by exercise, excitement, anger or even a pleasurable emotion.

ANGINA AND HEART ATTACKS

Being a born worrier, Peter wanted to know more about his angina. 'Is it serious?' he asked. 'Will it lead to a heart attack? What can be done to help it, and are there any other symptoms I should look out for?'

Angina is the name given to the chest pain that occurs when the coronary arteries are no longer able to provide enough blood to keep the heart muscles adequately oxygenated during exercise or emotion. This state of affairs is known as coronary insufficiency.

Anginal pain goes away once the patient rests. The chest pain, like that of a heart attack, is usually central or left-sided, and, also like that of a heart attack, it may radiate down the arms, particularly the left, into the neck and jaw (occasionally even into the nose) and sometimes into the thumb. Angina is often associated with a poor blood supply to the muscles of the calves of the legs so that when walking, particularly uphill or in a cold wind, sufferers have to stop regularly;

once they do, the leg pain disappears. The condition of the lower limb arteries which gives rise to this exercise-related pain is known medically as intermittent claudication.

Impotence, as the result of poor arterial blood supply to the penis, may be another early – sometimes first – warning sign of coronary arterial disease. Middle-aged men who are having trouble with increased impotence should have their coronary arteries investigated.

Angina is treated with glyceryl trinitrate, a tablet that is dissolved under the tongue. As it is absorbed, the coronary arteries dilate, the heart muscle has a better blood supply, and the pain disappears in a couple of minutes. There are other methods in which glyceryl trinitrate may be taken, including sprays, which are as rapidly absorbed.

If the coronary insufficiency is affecting the heart muscle so that it is no longer working as an efficient pump, the patient should also be taking an ACE inhibitor. There is evidence that this type of drug, which, among other actions, dilates blood vessels, helps to prolong life in a variety of ways.

The choice of beta blocker becomes most important once there is any evidence of heart strain, or early heart failure. Those that are alpha-beta blockers, such as Eucardic carvedilol, are indicated when there is heart failure, as a beta blocker that does not have the alpha-blocking component may increase the strain on the heart. These patients may also need a small dose of a diuretic drug (patients call them 'water pills'). At present, the standard diuretic drug used is bendrofluazide; note that no advantage is obtained from a diuretic by taking more than the prescribed dose.

Finally, any patient who is suffering from coronary arterial disease or who is at risk of cardiovascular disease should be taking one of the statin groups of drugs, even if their cholesterol level is normal. These not only lower cholesterol but make heart attacks, and some types of stroke, less likely.

Your cardiologist will decide what type of treatment you need after conducting a specialized examination of your heart arteries. This is done either with an angiogram (an X-ray of the coronary arteries), or possibly by means of a thalium scan, which will show how well the heart muscle is being supplied by blood.

The results of the examinations will determine whether any type of surgical intervention is necessary. This could include an angioplasty (a dilation of the blocked artery with a balloon) together with the fitting of stents (devices slipped into the artery to keep it open; stents may also be impregnated with a drug to prevent reclosure), or a bypass operation. In the latter, a blood vessel is taken from the chest (mediastinum) or the leg and used to replace the damaged vessel or vessels in the heart.

Recent research has shown that in the past in the UK, intervention – whether angioplasty or a bypass – has been delayed to the point of endangering patients' lives.

WHEN ANGINA CHANGES

Peter's next worry was what symptoms to watch out for that would show when his angina was crossing the barrier between being simply tiresome to being dangerous. His question: 'What are the changes in the nature of the pain which tell me I should consult my doctor immediately?'

The angina Peter has suffered is only slowly becoming more troublesome. This type of angina is referred to as stable angina, and it is unlikely to herald a disaster. The type and amount of exercise or emotion needed to bring on the anginal pain remains reasonably constant. It may vary according to the weather, whether or not food has been eaten recently, and other external factors such as tiredness and tension, but the amount of exercise needed to induce angina lessens only on a gradual basis.

The other type of angina is unstable angina. This constitutes an emergency, and it needs immediate treatment. Once a person's angina becomes unstable, its nature changes. The sufferer notices that, suddenly, the pain is induced much more readily; it may come on while at rest or even while the patient is in bed. As a result, the pain is not only more readily induced but it is more frequently induced. It may also last longer, be greater and may not always be so readily relieved by glycerol trinitrate (see page 21).

Once any of these changes have occurred, it is likely that a plaque of atheroma – the fatty material that collects in the arteries – has ruptured or become detached from the arterial wall. Consequently, the patient is very likely to suffer a heart attack in the near future. He or she should be admitted to hospital as soon as possible.

CORONARY HEART DISEASE

Peter's wife is as demanding in bed as she is around the house. Is it safe for him to respond to her advances? May he still visit the latest in his long line of women friends who help him forget his problems? Is the exertion of making love likely to be dangerous? Should he continue to take other exercise?

Whether or not they have had a heart attack, people who have been diagnosed with coronary arterial disease are helped by regular, steady (but not violent) aerobic exercise. They should take a brisk walk every day for not less than half an hour, and preferably for three-quarters of an hour. They should avoid this exercise only when the weather is extreme: either too hot, too humid or too cold, particularly if it is also windy.

The walking should be brisk enough for conversation to be possible, but talking should still be difficult. Violent exercise such as running, tennis, squash, skiing and any riding other than a gentle hack is not a good idea.

A British cardiological unit that made a

study of exercise and heart disease suggested to its patients a few years ago that the only exercise they should take was brisk walking or non-competitive bicycling. The researchers even had their doubts about swimming – unless it was warm, and the patient entered the pool slowly.

However, there is good news about sex. Evidence shows that it is unlikely for patients, male or female, to give up their sex lives because of heart disease, even if they have had a bypass operation. Dr Graham Jackson, a cardiologist at Guy's Hospital in London, has made a special study of exercise in heart disease, and from his survey he has found that the average lovemaking lasts for fifteen minutes, of which only three minutes are very intense. This is no longer than the time it takes to carry out an ECG (heart-tracing) stress test, so that if the patient's heart doesn't show unacceptable strain after that, then all should be well in bed.

Dr Jackson recommends an even simpler test than an ECG to judge the fitness of a heart for sex. The stress on the heart during intercourse is equivalent to walking up twenty-six standard household stairs in ten seconds, or walking one mile on level ground in twenty minutes. If neither of these tasks cause problems, then neither will sex.

Peter may have one disappointment in store. Most doctors try to discourage extra-marital sex in heart patients, because sex with new (or comparatively new) partners causes more stress and a greater increase in blood pressure than marital sex. Death among coronary heart disease sufferers occurs more frequently when they have intercourse with casual or new partners rather than with their husbands or wives. The other situation that may trigger trouble is sex after a heavy meal, typically during siesta time on holiday. When sex is abandoned on health grounds, it is most commonly because of arthritis – not because of heart disease.

WHAT IS A HEART ATTACK?

Peter next asked a question that concerns not only him, but nearly everyone diagnosed with angina. 'What do people mean by "having a heart attack"?' he wondered. 'How do I know if I have had one, and what should I do if I do?'

I often meet people who tell me that they have had a heart attack. Heart attack and coronary thrombosis are the popular terms for the condition doctors describe as a myocardial infarction, or MI.

During a heart attack, the myocardium, or heart muscle, is suddenly deprived of life-preserving oxygen and other nutrients carried by the blood as a result of one of the coronary arteries becoming blocked, usually by a clot. Consequently, the area of muscle supplied by the blocked artery dies; technically, it has become 'infarcted' (withered and dead): hence the medical term 'myocardial infarction'. Eventually, the dead muscle is replaced by scar tissue.

If a patient dies, it is usually because the

heart attack has triggered a fatal arrhythmia (abnormal heartbeat); it is only occasionally the direct result of too large a portion of the heart muscle being destroyed. The need to reduce the irritability of the heart muscle, and hence its liability to develop a potentially fatal arrhythmia, is one good reason why patients with coronary heart disease should take a beta blocker and stop smoking.

The symptoms of a heart attack are similar to those of angina, but they last longer and are associated with shock. Medical shock is not the same as the surprise, anxiety and anguish described as shock by the popular press. Clinical shock describes the condition in which a person is collapsed, feels faint, is sweating, nauseated (even vomiting) and has a grey, damp complexion accompanied by a feeble pulse and a low blood pressure.

Although the chest pain associated with a heart attack is usually crippling, in a fifth of cases it is either mild or even absent. The usual pain may be often felt right across the chest. It is, as patients tell their doctors, as if someone has dropped a sack of cement on their ribs. Other patients describe it as like having a band slowly tightened around the chest, just as if the chest were a beer barrel and the cooper were tightening the metal strips around it.

Whatever the pain's exact nature, patients experience the sensation that they can't breathe and that the Grim Reaper is already hovering over them. Sometimes the full force of the pain is not felt immediately but works up to a peak. As in angina, pain may radiate down one or both arms (usually the left), into the upper back, or up into the neck and even the jaw.

The severity of the pain depends on the size of the artery that is blocked and the amount of heart muscle that has been starved of blood and oxygen. Unlike angina, however, the pain, when it occurs, is not relieved by the under-the-tongue tablets or sprays that contain glycerol trinitrate. Also unlike angina, it isn't eased by rest; it lasts for at least half an hour, and usually for very much longer.

Some heart attacks, in which a small artery is blocked, may cause such slight pain that they are confused with indigestion. These could be classified as 'silent' heart attacks: ones that are painless or near-painless.

Once someone has had a heart attack, the immediate first-aid response should be to give him or her an aspirin. All patients at risk of heart attacks should always carry aspirins with them. They should have one beside their beds, along with some water, another in the locker of their car dashboard, and one on their person.

The next step is to call 999 and describe the symptoms. Paramedics are trained to deal with heart attacks. They are empowered to administer on-the-spot clot-busting drugs, and they carry a defibrillator: a machine used to treat potentially fatal arrhythmia.

Heart failure

Mrs Wilkinson is over sixty-five and has many features typical of people who develop heart failure. She is overweight, and for many years has had raised blood pressure that has been inadequately treated. She also has minor angina when exercising. Recently, she has become increasingly breathless and her feet have begun to swell. Her question is very much to the point. 'I'm told I have heart failure,' she says. 'Does this mean I am likely to drop dead?'

Mrs Wilkinson is not likely to drop dead. Even so, her condition needs skilled and vigorous treatment or it will limit both the quality of her life and its length. Heart failure is a frightening term used by doctors that is often misunderstood by patients. In the past, some doctors even preferred to call heart failure 'heart strain'. They thought that this was both less misleading and less disturbing.

Heart failure simply means that, because of the deterioration in the heart muscle, the pumping action of the heart is no longer powerful enough to keep all of the body's essential organs supplied with oxygen and nutrients. Even the smartest and fastest cars' engines become slower and feebler with the years. Likewise, the heart muscle becomes weaker with time, or – less often in younger people – as the result of various heart diseases.

The most common cause of heart failure is coronary arterial disease and its associated high blood pressure, which lead to the heart muscle having a poor blood supply and inadequate oxygen. High blood pressure not only predisposes people to coronary arterial disease, but it puts an increased load on the heart muscle – a load that may cause premature wear. The pumping action of the heart will also be strained if the valves between its pumping chambers either leak or are too tight (stenosed).

Sometimes the progress of heart failure can be prevented or slowed by coronary bypass surgery, angioplasty, or valvular heart surgery (see page 23), but bypass surgery and angioplasty can sometimes make the situation worse in patients whose heart muscle is very frail and feeble. The principal treatment of heart failure is via medication, yet heart failure is very undertreated; too often this leads to an unnecessarily miserable and restricted old age, and an even shorter life.

If anyone is diagnosed with high blood pressure, it should be reduced to normal levels. Patients should be dissuaded from smoking or drinking to excess, and they should diet so that they are not overweight – even if, as Mrs Wilkinson has discovered, this is difficult.

Usually, a combination of drugs is used to treat heart failure. Increasingly, doctors are realizing that, to achieve the best control, it will probably be necessary to prescribe more than one type of tablet or pill daily. Most patients with heart failure are prescribed a diuretic such as bendrofluazide, an ACE inhibitor (often Tritace ramipril) and an alpha-beta blocker such as Eucardic carvedilol. Anyone when first beginning treatment with alpha-beta blockers requires expert supervision.

Palpitations

Life as a receptionist in a large hotel is one of constant stress – as Jane, who works in one, has discovered. Travellers are tense and anxious and take out any frustrations or worries over their schedule on the staff behind the desk. Recently, Jane has had palpitations. She asks if she should be worried. The hotel doctor has patted her on the back, told her not to worry and that she will probably live to be a hundred.

The term 'palpitations' means no more than an abnormal awareness of the heartbeat. This may be because the rhythm of the heart is irregular or because it is too fast. It may be related to the position in which a person is sitting or lying; some people become alarmed when they are conscious of their heart as they lie in bed at night. Before reassuring Jane, the hotel doctor probably took her pulse, blood pressure and listened to the heart, and in all likelihood carried out an ECG (heart-tracing test).

Doctors routinely order blood tests for a

patient with palpitations to exclude any anaemias and an over-active thyroid. If all these tests were normal, and as one of the commonest causes of palpitations – stress – is obviously present, Jane's doctor's reassurance was justified.

In older people, and in those with a less obvious cause of palpitations, other possibilities need exclusion. Increasingly, doctors are using a Holter mobile ECG recorder (monitor) to take recordings of the heart's rhythm and rate over a long period of time.

Many people have extra systoles (ectopic beats): momentary abnormal rhythms of the heartbeat. Instead of the usual regular beat, there is an early beat followed by a pause, and after the pause, a beat that is stronger than usual, and the patient notices it.

Extra systoles are the most common cause of palpitations and are usually quite harmless. They may be related to stress, and also to too much tea or coffee.

A heart that is beating too fast, or 'racing' as many patients say, is also commonly described as palpitations. A heart rate that is greater than normal is known medically as tachycardia. This occurs naturally when someone is exercising or when a person becomes excited, but it may also be associated with anaemia, an over-active thyroid gland, fevers or (more rarely) some other illness. Other types of cardiac arrhythmias (abnormal heartbeats) may also induce tachycardia.

Bradycardia, which is the medical term for an abnormally slow heartbeat, is found in athletes and in others who take a great deal of exercise. It may, however, also be a symptom of a heart block; sick sinus disease, when there is trouble with the part of the heart from which the beat originates; and other abnormalities of the conducting system of the heart. These conditions can result in periods of dizziness, faintness or even unconsciousness, and they need investigation by a doctor. On occasion, a pacemaker will be fitted in order to regulate the beat.

Atrial fibrillation is a very common cause of palpitations in older people, or in younger people who have suffered heart disease. When the heart is fibrillating, which is a rapid, chaotic and uncoordinated beating of individual muscle fibres, the atria, or collecting chambers of the heart, beat irregularly in an uncoordinated fashion – so irregularly, in fact, that they no longer act as an efficient pump. The heartbeat is rapid and irregularly irregular. As the circulation is no longer being driven effectively, patients become breathless, tire easily and may even develop angina or dizziness. They will complain of palpitations.

Efforts are made to persuade the patient's runaway heart rhythm to return to normal by administering an electric shock (defibrillation). If it is impossible to restore a normal rhythm in this way, drugs may be necessary to control the heart rate. In patients who are fibrillating, anticoagulants are always prescribed to reduce the risk of stroke. Investigations are necessary to see if there is any treatable underlying cause for the fibrillation.

Hypertension

Roger was an overweight country solicitor: hard-working, conscientious, under-exercised and, in his family's opinion, underpaid. He was puzzled. 'I have been told that I have hypertension,' he said. 'I always thought hypertension was something that affected tetchy, red-faced, choleric colonels. What exactly is hypertension?'

Contrary to widespread belief, hypertension has nothing to do with a short temper, intolerance, or red, weather-beaten faces. Hypertension is simply the medical term for high blood pressure.

There is always a constant pressure exerted by the elasticity of the arteries on the blood within them; otherwise, when the heart wasn't beating, the brain and other essential organs would immediately be deprived of a blood supply. In essence, the blood pressure is related to the force, or pressure, which a beating heart exerts to circulate the blood around the body.

When the heart contracts, the blood pressure

rises; this is the systolic pressure and the first reading given by doctors. When the heart is relaxing, the pressure in the arteries falls; this is the diastolic blood pressure, the second reading recorded by the doctor. The aim is to keep the blood pressure with a systolic below 140, the diastolic below 90 – this would be expressed as 140 over 90. Advancing years is no reason to tolerate raised blood pressure, although it may be more difficult to keep the blood pressure down.

Mild, even moderate high blood pressure has no symptoms. By the time raised blood pressure has caused headaches, blurred vision, nosebleeds, extreme tiredness, breathlessness or other signs of heart failure such as swollen feet, it is already well-established and may have done irreparable harm. Everyone over forty should have an annual blood pressure check.

Left untreated, high blood pressure increases the chance of a stroke: a haemorrhage in the brain or the obstruction of one of the arteries in the brain. Seven out of ten people who have a stroke have raised blood pressure. It triples the likelihood that a person will have a heart attack, and experts have reckoned that high blood pressure is responsible for a third of all heart disease.

High blood pressure is less likely to affect people who take regular, steady exercise and who don't become overweight. Smoking is a serious risk factor – not only for coronary heart disease, but also for high blood pressure. Reducing the amount of salt in the diet, including the 'invisible' salt found in convenience foods, would help to reduce the prevalence of heart disease and high blood pressure. People of all ages should have their blood pressure taken regularly; those over forty should have it done annually.

Regimes that reduce high blood pressure also help reduce the incidence and prevalence of coronary arterial disease. Weight reduction; regular (but not violent) exercise; a diet in which animal fats are reduced to a point where they don't cause an unacceptably high level of cholesterol – in particular the low-density lipoprotein (LDL) cholesterol; no smoking; and alcohol (particularly red wine) in moderation are the essential features of a heart-friendly lifestyle.

No salt should be added to food while cooking, or when it is at the table. The diet should include oily fish at least twice a week, as well as plenty of fruit and vegetables that are rich in antioxidants. The desirable options include tomatoes, citrus fruits, red and green peppers, carrots, broccoli and in general all those fruits and vegetables that are brightly coloured. Lettuce, which figures so widely in restaurant salads, is virtually useless as a food, and is nothing more than an expensive way of buying water. Eat lettuce and enjoy it, but don't count it as a food that will contribute to health.

LOOK OUT FOR

Early Signs of Lung Cancer

increased breathlessness

worsening cough

increased phlegm

blood-speckled phlegm

a cough that doesn't respond to antibiotics

a cold, or flu, which 'hangs on'

any wheeze

Signs of Pneumonia in the Elderly

as well as increased breathlessness
and painful cough:

fatigue

confusion

dementia

a high temperature may be absent

3
HUFFERS & PUFFERS
Chest Diseases

Asthma

With two huge brown eyes set in a sensitive face that was surrounded by dark, curly hair, three-year-old Thomas looked like a Botticelli angel. His mother had been to the doctor to discuss her next pregnancy when she mentioned, as if by chance, that Thomas had developed a habit of coughing at night. She wondered if his recent cold had left him with chronic bronchitis.

The doctor asked Thomas's mother to bring him round to the surgery the next time he was ill. Sure enough, when the little boy breathed deeply, there was an audible wheeze. A golden rule of medicine is that a child who wheezes has asthma until it is proved otherwise. Indeed, asthma should be considered as a possible diagnosis in anyone who wheezes, whatever the age group.

The symptoms characteristic of asthma are wheezing, breathlessness, chest tightness and a dry cough, which is often only noticeable at nights. The child is sometimes as bright as a button during the day and cough-free. Asthma with wheezing and a protracted nocturnal cough often follows a cough and cold, just as it had done in Thomas's case. It may also be triggered by various allergens, including house mites, some moulds, animal dandruff or saliva, some foods, and strenuous exercise, particularly in the cold air.

Indeed, cold air may be enough to precipitate an attack even in the absence of exercise. Older children or adults notice that exercise, when it is competitive and strenuous, may not cause an immediate asthma attack, but its symptoms may come on once they are relaxing and recovering after a race or game. Pollution may not often be the basic cause of asthma, but once it has taken hold, pollution may, and often does, trigger attacks.

Aspirin (which wouldn't apply to Thomas as children under sixteen should never be given aspirin) or other anti-inflammatory drugs, beta blockers, and some of the drugs used to treat bladder troubles may also induce an attack of asthma. There may be evidence of other allergen-induced conditions, and there is often a family history. Although domestic tension, increased emotion, and stress may make asthma attacks more likely, asthmatic patients are not more highly strung than their contemporaries.

Asthma can start at any age. The symptoms may vary in intensity between attacks, and even during an attack. The frequency of attacks is not necessarily related to their severity, but any patient of whatever age should have specialist advice so that the patient, the GP and the specialist can agree on a plan of campaign together. Once this has been established, the asthma becomes much better controlled because, if there is an acute severe attack, the patient knows just when to go into hospital in order to receive potentially life-saving treatment.

Thomas's parents may well find that his symptoms become so severe that when there is an attack, breathing is difficult and his tummy becomes drawn in beneath the ribs with each breath. Luckily, as a child grows older, asthma usually improves and often disappears.

Because everyone concerned now makes

detailed plans as to how to deal with attacks, and access to hospitals is faster and easier, the death rate from asthma in the UK has tumbled.

Many asthmatic children may also suffer from allergies. Particular care should be taken to avoid exposure to nuts, especially peanuts, which may sensitize allergy-prone children to nut allergy.

In the event of anybody, child or adult, who has displayed an allergic response to any particular substance, whether eggs, nuts, bee or wasp stings or even medications (including aspirin and antibiotics), every effort must be taken to avoid them. If they have ever shown signs of hypersensitivity – nettle-type rash, swollen face and eyes, difficulty in breathing (from the constriction of mouth and throat), palpitations, and later, nausea, vomiting and collapse – they should always carry adrenaline (Epipen).

BREATHLESSNESS

Sid Brown, the local gravedigger and church caretaker, was never without a cigarette. Short and wiry, he could be seen striding to the churchyard, a pick, spade and shovel over his shoulders. Friends noticed that his walk was slowing and he was taking longer to dig a grave. Finally, he had to admit it: not only was the gravedigging becoming too much for him, he even found it difficult to climb the church stairs to wind the clock. He was unusually tired and breathless, and his cough, a nuisance for years during the winter, now lasted the whole year long. Sid wondered whether his increased breathlessness was related to smoking, or if there were some other cause – heart failure, for instance?

Doctors ask patients very carefully about the way in which breathlessness has developed. They want to know if it is of sudden onset, coming on within a matter of days, has taken weeks to develop, or is of the type that has been slowly increasing for years, creeping up on patients so insidiously that they have barely noticed its progress.

Sid's breathlessness fell into the last group. As he had done a job requiring hard physical exercise, he had noticed his increasing shortness of breath rather earlier than would have been the case had he worked in an office. The reason was obvious: Sid had smoked forty home-rolled cigarettes a day, and his childhood, spent in a damp cottage, had been tough and hard. He was now paying the penalty for his adult addiction to tobacco, as well as for his early surroundings over which he had no control.

Sid had chronic bronchitis and emphysema. Chronic bronchitis results in inflammation and swelling of the lining of the tubes, known as the bronchi, which lead to the lungs. Although in Sid's case, the damage to the bronchi was started by the irritation caused by tobacco smoke, recurrent infections add to it. The lungs are like a pair of sponges composed of many air sacs. In emphysema, these sacs become damaged and enlarged, and as they enlarge there is less lung tissue available through which oxygen may be absorbed. As a result, patients become breathless.

Chronic bronchitis and emphysema are now known by many chest physicians as chronic obstructive pulmonary disease, or COPD. In COPD, the cough is classically productive of phlegm, initially copious but grey, later yellow or even green. When the chest troubles are beginning, the cough occurs during the three winter months; later it may extend throughout the year. Chronic bronchitis is only diagnosed, and labelled as such by doctors, once the patient has suffered it during two consecutive years.

The change in colour of the phlegm from dirty grey to yellow or green shows the presence of a secondary infection. The cough is often associated with a wheeze, which makes a mis-diagnosis of asthma possible. The symptom of breathlessness, as in Sid's case, advances very slowly in its early stages, more rapidly when the patient is middle-aged or older. This enables patients, and sometimes their doctors, to dismiss it all too easily as a normal effect of ageing. It isn't. Breathlessness always needs an explanation, however old the person may be.

The damage already done by forty years of smoking and the recurrent childhood infections in a cold, damp house cannot be reversed. The object of treatment in any case is to halt or slow further deterioration in the bronchi and the lungs. Patients should be spared further exposure to dust, smoke (Sid will have to give up his cigarettes) and inclement weather.

Increasingly, treatments are available which will ease the symptoms of COPD, allowing the person to continue as normal for many years longer than was previously possible.

Anyone with COPD should always have anti-flu jabs and should be immunized against pneumococcal pneumonia.

CANCER OF THE LUNG

Margaret is in her late seventies. The high point of her life was her time as a Wren during the war, when she served with a motor torpedo boat unit in Dorset. The men were glamorous, the job exciting, but she often had time on her hands when all she could do was sit around, smoking and chatting. By the time Margaret left the navy, she was an addicted smoker. When she went to see the doctor, her question was simple: why was she losing weight?

Like most heavy smokers, Margaret had had what she liked to refer to as a 'smoker's cough' for so long – more than half a century, in fact – that she hadn't noticed that it was gradually becoming worse, and that her breathlessness was increasing. Whatever other symptoms people with lung cancer (which was Margaret's trouble) have, it is only in exceptional circumstances that they don't develop a cough and increased breathlessness. In most cases, there is also an increase in the amount of phlegm produced, and this may be streaked with blood. However, it is a common error to think that if there is no blood, there is no cancer; bleeding may, in some types of tumour, be a late sign.

If patients like Margaret are already suffering from chronic bronchitis – a more honest but harsher term for 'smoker's cough' – the cough will become worse once a cancer develops. Also, a patient's attention is often drawn to the possibility of cancer by an increase in breathlessness, a worsening cough or the presence of blood. Later, there is often an associated loss of weight, a loss of appetite, and sometimes chest pain or a hoarseness of the voice. Other sufferers may notice that their chest symptoms are accompanied by additional problems such as fatigue, loss of enthusiasm, weakness and sometimes fever.

The real tragedy is that, even in the best units, cancer of the lung – which in eighty-seven percent of cases is related to smoking – is often only diagnosed after it is already incurable. The objective of doctors today is to achieve earlier diagnosis. Improved methods of X-raying chests will help achieve this, but it is expected that a greater advance will be made when patients, particularly those who are or who have been smokers, can be persuaded to visit their doctors at an earlier stage of the disease.

Warning symptoms for lung cancer include any change for the worse in a cough or breathlessness, or any alteration in the nature or quantity of the phlegm produced, including streaking with blood. In particular, patients are asked to report to their surgeries if an ordinary winter cough, cold or attack of flu hangs on for more than a couple of weeks, or hasn't responded as completely or as quickly as usual to antibiotics.

Attacks of pneumonia and pleurisy should always be viewed with suspicion and need careful investigation by a doctor, both when first diagnosed and during any follow-up sessions.

Tuberculosis

Sam was a disappointment to his parents, yet they remained loyal and, as he grew older, hid their dismay that he had left his university course to become a freelance musician. Sam lived a hand-to-mouth existence in tatty, crowded and damp lodgings and travelled extensively. He drank to excess and smoked tobacco and cannabis. Sam's symptoms – cough, night sweats, loss of weight and breathlessness – were not a surprise, but the diagnosis took his doctor, as well as his family, unawares.

Sam had had a perpetual snuffly nose and cough for as long as anyone could remember; indeed, he hadn't looked healthy – or even reasonably fed – since he had left school. Hence the lack of surprise when his cough worsened, and he became thinner and even more languorous than ever. He felt awful. At last he went to his doctor. 'Am I ill,' he asked, 'or is it just my lifestyle?'

The doctor asked all the usual questions and discovered that Sam's cough had been growing more troublesome for the past six months, ever since he had returned from the Far East. Sam agreed when it was suggested that he was using rather more cannabis than he used to. As it happens, cannabis is even more of an irritant than undiluted tobacco smoke.

The cough was productive and associated with a bit of the wheeze, and Sam told the doctor that he thought that he had had several attacks of 'flu' over the past few months. He certainly knew that he had had a temperature and was having night sweats. He was thinner than ever and was now beginning to wonder just how he could keep going.

The doctor diagnosed chronic bronchitis in a heavy smoker who was also chronically undernourished. As Sam was breathless and wheezy, his doctor thought there might also be an asthmatic component to his chest troubles.

Sam was treated for some months with a variety of antibiotics, yet when he not only failed to show progress but was becoming so emaciated as to be as wasted as a famine victim, he was sent to a chest clinic.

Sam was diagnosed with tuberculosis, or TB. TB characteristically (but not exclusively) affects the homeless, alcoholics and drug users, drifters and those persons who are mentally or psychologically compromised. People who hail from or have visited countries where the disease is more common than in the UK are also at increased risk of catching TB.

Sam did very well. When it came to following instructions essential for his recovery, he cooperated fully during the six-month course of treatment. During that time, his doctors rang the changes with the various antibiotics available.

There is one danger in telling Sam's story, and that is that not everyone suffering from tuberculosis shows such an obvious case history. The most hard-working, abstemious, clean-living, ordered, continent person may unwittingly become a contact and catch TB. Anyone with shortness of breath, an inexplicable cough lasting more than two or three weeks (only in late TB is the sputum usually blood-stained), fever, night sweats and tiredness should seek medical attention.

LOOK OUT FOR

Signs of Upper Gastro-Intestinal Cancers
worsening indigestion that is not relieved by antacids

loss of appetite

bloating

sense of fullness after a small meal

any difficulty in swallowing

sensation that food is sticking

loss of weight

unexplained fatigue

any vomiting of blood

black, sticky bowel motions

Signs of Gall-Bladder Problems
upper abdominal pain

jaundice (yellow tint to skin and whites of eyes;
brownish urine; pale, clay-coloured bowel motions)

4
REPEATS & RETURNS
Upper Gastro-Intestinal Disease

Abdominal pain and cancer

Trevor is a sixty-year-old builder. These days, his business concentrates mostly on painting and decorating. He is hard-working but always finds time to enjoy a drink with his colleagues at the local pub after work. He smokes up to twenty cigarettes a day. The thirty-one-inch waist he boasted in his twenties has ballooned to forty-one inches. For years, Trevor has had epigastric pain – pain in the pit of his stomach – which is increasingly less easily controlled with antacids such as Rennies. Food no longer eases it, and he sometimes suffers nausea after a meal. Recently, and for the first time in forty years, he has had to take in a notch on his belt. His appetite is reduced, as he is readily satisfied by his food, and he tires more quickly. Once or twice he has not even felt like joining his team at the George and Dragon after work.

Although cancers of the oesophagus are more common, those of the stomach are now less frequently seen, and there has been a shift in the part of the stomach that is usually involved.

This may well be the result of the discovery of the importance played by the Helicobacter pylori bacterium in stomach and duodenal ulcers and of the means to eradicate it.

It is not yet proved, but very possibly some of the changes in the incidence of cancer of the stomach may stem from the greater use of the proton-pump inhibitors, the most effective drugs prescribed for the reduction of gastric acidity, such as Losec omeprazole or Nexium esomeprazole. These and the other drugs of this group have revolutionized the treatment of dyspepsia indigestion.

The cause of Trevor's condition is difficult to diagnose, and can only be determined after a thorough investigation with X-rays and an endoscope. This illuminated fibre-optic tube enables a doctor to view the inside of a person's stomach and guts (gastro-intestinal tract).

The early symptoms of early cancer of the stomach depend on the part of the stomach that is affected; initially, symptoms may not be troublesome. A cancer situated high in the stomach may mimic oesophagitis (inflammation of the gullet; see page 17). Tumours located in other parts of it may cause pain very similar to that of a gastric ulcer. The pain is situated high in the mid-line of the abdomen, but it responds less well (if at all) to the medication prescribed for indigestion and ulcer pain. Unlike ulcer pain, it is not relieved by eating.

The traditional belief that stomach cancer frequently starts as a chronic gastric ulcer is no longer thought to be true. If this does happen, it is only an occasional occurrence.

Initially, cancer of the stomach produces few, if any, generalized symptoms, but in time ulcer-type pain, a loss of appetite and a sense of fullness after eating only a small meal become obvious. This bloating and 'satiety', a sense of early fullness when eating, not necessarily accompanied by pain, are early symptoms, but they are too frequently ignored.

Stomach cancers bleed, and as a result, the patient will usually become anaemic and tired. If there is a considerable haemorrhage, patients may either vomit blood or pass black, sticky stools. Vomit after bleeding into the stomach doesn't always look blood-stained but may be brown and resemble coffee grounds.

Weight loss is a common symptom in cancer of the stomach, but it is often a patient's family and friends who first notice that he or she is tired and listless and is losing weight. A strange feature of cancer of the stomach is that it is unusual to find it in people who have a long history of duodenal pain or ulceration. Cancer of the duodenum itself is very rare and never starts as a duodenal ulcer.

Difficulty swallowing

Justin, aged sixty-six, is a retired journalist of the old school. He had enjoyed every minute of the hurly-burly of the newsdesk. He also enjoyed even more the camaraderie that went with it – another way of saying that Justin had, in fact, smoked and drunk too much all his working life. His question, more of a statement, rang the loudest of alarm bells: 'Doctor, I can't swallow properly.'

This statement always arouses immediate concern because it is often the first symptom that draws a person's attention to a cancer in the oesophagus. A doctor can immediately exclude acute infective causes of swallowing difficulties such as tonsillitis, peritonsular abscesses (quinsies) and pharyngitis (inflammation of the pharynx, or throat), which lie higher in the neck. They usually respond to antibiotic treatment (although quinsy may need minor surgery) and the alarm is over. Once it becomes likely that the difficulty in swallowing stems from the oesophagus, there is anxiety until the cause has been shown not to be malignant.

Initially, patients with an obstruction in their oesophagus find it difficult to swallow solid foods, particularly pieces of meat or bread. Later, sloppy foods create problems, and finally, even fluids. Early cancers of the oesophagus give rise neither to pain nor to problems with eating. When such cancers are larger, there may be pain as well as discomfort on swallowing, and the pain may radiate through to the back.

Even as Justin was talking, his doctor was looking at his collar and judging how loose it was. Patients lose weight with a cancer of the oesophagus even before they have noticed that swallowing is becoming difficult. As one would expect, other symptoms are general weight loss, anaemia and a loss of vitality. Less common symptoms may include pressure on the nerves that lead to the vocal cords so that the person's voice progressively becomes more hoarse. Occasionally, involvement of another nerve in the neck may lead to changes in the size of the pupils and the way they react to light.

Because early diagnosis is the only path to

a successful treatment, doctors are always on the lookout for this cancer. Fortunately, a large number of benign problems may cause some difficulty in swallowing. Some patients, usually young women who are over-stressed, over-tense and anxious, develop a feeling that something is stuck in their throat and that they will choke. While this can never be dismissed without X-ray and endoscopy examination, the patient's personality and inability to point precisely to where the food is sticking usually provide clues as to the true diagnosis.

Another fairly common cause of difficulty in swallowing is oesophagitis (see page 17), which can, if it is a long-standing condition, lead to scarring and narrowing of the oesophagus. In other cases, achalasia, which is a spasm in the oesophageal muscles, causes obstruction.

GALL-BLADDER PROBLEMS

Suzanne is short, fair, rather overweight and forty-three. She answers the description every medical student has been taught is typical of a patient who has gall-bladder disease. Not surprisingly, Suzanne wants to know if the upper abdominal pain she is experiencing, particularly after eating fatty foods, is indeed coming from her gall-bladder.

Like most aphorisms, the belief that gall-bladder disease affects only the short, fat, fair and forty-something female is both misleading and a gross over-simplification. However, there is enough truth in it so that when Suzanne complained of pain in her upper right abdomen beneath the ribs which became worse when she breathed in, and told her doctor that the pain radiated to her right shoulder, the diagnosis was obvious.

There is debate as to whether gall-bladder symptoms are made worse, as has been believed for centuries, by eating fatty foods. The pain from the gall-bladder, if stones are present, is often colicky in nature. If the patient becomes jaundiced, the urine dark brown and the motions clay-coloured because a gall-stone has become stuck in the common bile duct, the likely diagnosis is obvious.

More often, patients who are later found to have gall-bladder disease initially have no more than vague symptoms of recurrent attacks of nausea, vomiting and a loss of appetite, together with some upper-abdominal discomfort and tenderness when the abdomen is felt – much less clearly defined symptoms than Suzanne's.

As ten percent of people have gall-stones without experiencing any symptoms from them at all, it is difficult to know if these ill-defined symptoms, allegedly worse after fatty foods, are as good diagnostic pointers to gall-bladder disease as was once thought.

When a diseased gall-bladder gives rise to symptoms, the treatment of choice is a cholecystectomy, or the surgical removal of the gall-bladder. This is performed either by the standard method, which involves a wide incision below the right ribs, or by laparoscopic (keyhole) surgery.

Various medications have been given to treat gall-stones. These will dissolve some types of stones, but since the underlying reason for their initial formation hasn't been removed, the weeks or months of treatment needed to dissolve them are usually followed, depressingly soon, by the formation of new ones.

Like most people who have gall-bladder disease, Suzanne wanted to know whether, if she didn't have surgery, she would be at risk of developing gall-bladder cancer. Although still rare, this cancer and cancer of the bile duct are some of the tumours which, for reasons as yet unknown, are becoming more common. There is therefore a risk, but it is a very small one.

The greater risk for those not having a diseased gall-bladder removed is that severe inflammation, known as cholecystitis, may occur when the person concerned is in some far corner of the world where skilled surgical attention is not readily available.

GORD

Mr Adam Donovan's question was one that might have been asked by forty-five percent of the adult population. Like four percent of all those who attend their GP's surgeries, Adam complained of heartburn and acid regurgitation. 'After I go to bed at night,' he explained, 'or if I stoop during the day, as for instance when gardening, or after a heavy meal, I suffer severe indigestion with a burning sensation that rises from my stomach into my upper chest and then into the throat. I can feel the acid in my gullet.'

If patients suffer from these symptoms more than twice a week, the likely diagnosis is something called gastro-oesophageal reflux disease, often referred to as GORD for short. GORD is the technical term for the severe indigestion that people experience when the acidic contents of the stomach 'reflux', or flow back, from the stomach into the oesophagus (the gullet).

The lining of the stomach is designed to

withstand acids, but when the stomach acids reach the oesophagus, its lining is quite unprepared to receive them. As a result, the burning acid may at first induce irritation, followed later by inflammation of the gullet (oesophagitis), and finally, sometimes by scarring. These symptoms may cause difficulty or discomfort in swallowing.

The reflux into the throat of stomach acids may allow acidic fumes to rise to the larynx, where they can cause a husky voice from inflammation of the vocal cords. The pain of oesophagitis may not only be felt high in the central chest area, but, just like angina, it may also radiate down the arms and up into the neck. The pain may be very severe.

Although people always think of acid regurgitation as being related to an excess of acids in the stomach, this is not strictly so. The problem arises when the acid is in the wrong place, because the sphincter that separates the oesophagus and stomach is not tight enough, and the acidic stomach contents are able to flow into the bottom end of the oesophagus. A sphincter is a ring of muscle that surrounds an orifice.

Chronic oesophagitis may also lead to ulceration and, very occasionally, bleeding. In a minority of patients, chronic inflammation of the lining of the oesophagus may result in changes in its cells, giving rise to what is known as a Barratt's oesophagus. In a small minority of those with cases of Barratt's oesophagus, these changes later lead to cancer of the oesophagus.

Just as with simple forms of indigestion, losing weight, reducing alcohol intake and giving up smoking are laudable aims. These will make some difference to the obese, as well as to heavy drinkers and smokers, but, unlike Adam Donovan, more than two-thirds of patients with GORD drink little, do not smoke and have a normal girth. Apart from changes in lifestyle, the treatment is to alter the acidity of the stomach contents or else to reduce the production of acid within the stomach itself.

Antacids such as Rennie Duo provide excellent short-term relief. For longer-term treatment, either H_2 receptor antagonists (for example, Tagamet cimetidine or Zantac ranitidine) or a proton pump inhibitor such as Losec or Nexium are necessary (see page 63).

Improved medication has reduced the need for surgery to prevent reflux. Anyone who has persistent simple indigestion or GORD that has lasted for even a few weeks despite treatment should seek medical attention.

Peptic ulcers

Hamish Murray – tall, thin, and with a face as humourless and sour as his stomach contents – is a lifelong sufferer from indigestion. A couple of hours after a meal, he develops pain between his belly button and his lower ribs. The pain is relieved by taking Rennie Duos. Hamish has been reading the popular papers and wants to know whether what he has always thought of as simple indigestion is, in fact, pain from an ulcer.

The outlook for people who have either a stomach ulcer or a duodenal ulcer, from which Mr Murray may well be suffering, has been revolutionized since 1994. Then it became accepted that stomach and duodenal ulcers were usually related to the presence in the stomach of a bacterium known as Helicobacter pylori. Not everybody who has Helicobacter pylori has ulcers, but the majority of people who have ulcers can be cured by ridding the body of this organism.

As a result of finding ways to eradicate

Helicobacter pylori, the days when the ulcer sufferer was treated with tranquilizers and lectured on stress, lack of sleep and a faulty diet, and was given gallons of indigestion medicine have gone. There are different regimes for the eradication of Helicobacter pylori which use different types of gastric-acid suppressants and various antibiotics for different lengths of time. The most successful regimes will eradicate the bacterium in over ninety percent of cases. Once the patients' stomachs are rid of this corkscrew-shaped pest, their ulcers are cured.

The presence of Helicobacter pylori can be confirmed either by a blood test, which looks for antibodies produced as a reaction to it; by a breath test in which the breath is analyzed after swallowing a particular chemical; or by taking a sample from the stomach lining by endoscopy. Hamish Murray's symptoms were typical of someone with a duodenal ulcer.

The pain is felt in the upper abdomen, usually slightly to the right of the mid-line. The painful area is also tender, and hurts when the doctor presses it. By day, the pain usually starts mid-morning. It is relieved by eating at lunch but occurs two or three hours after food. It is also eased by antacids, but is apt to wake the patient in the middle of the night – hence the bottles of indigestion medicine and Rennies by the bed.

A gastric ulcer – that is, an ulcer eroding the lining of the stomach – has less clearly defined symptoms than a duodenal ulcer. The pain from it, as from a duodenal ulcer, is mainly felt in the epigastrium, the area between the belly button and the breast bone, but the pain from a gastric ulcer tends to be more mid-line than that from the duodenum. Gastric ulcer pain doesn't have such a definite relation to food; it can either be made better or worse by eating, whereas patients with a duodenal ulcer usually find that eating eases it.

Two common complications of ulceration are perforation or haemorrhage. When an ulcer perforates, it has penetrated the whole thickness of the stomach or duodenal wall. This causes the contents of the gut to spill out into the abdominal cavity, where they cause irritation, very severe pain associated with shock and collapse, and a potentially fatal peritonitis.

After bleeding (haemorrhage) from an ulcer, the patient may vomit blood, which may be red and fresh, or dark brown (like coffee grounds) because it has partly digested. If the patient doesn't vomit blood, the blood passes through the gut and turns the motions black and sticky.

Both ulcerative haemorrhage and perforation are surgical emergencies that need immediate treatment and hospitalization.

Patients who have peptic ulceration (whether gastric or duodenal ulceration) or chronic indigestion, should avoid taking aspirin and other anti-inflammatory drugs, without first consulting their doctors. This precaution is particularly important in people over the age of sixty-five.

LOOK OUT FOR

Early Signs of Cancer of the Colon and Rectum

any change in bowel habits

constipation, diarrhoea or an apparent
mixture of both

change in the consistency of bowel motions

change in shape of bowel motions
('boot-lace' motions)

passing any blood, or blood-flecked motions

lower abdominal pain or discomfort

loss of weight

increasing and unusual fatigue

5
WASTE DISPOSAL
Lower Gastro-Intestinal Disease

Rectal bleeding

Paul Harrison was a seventy-year-old retired bank manager. After going to the lavatory one morning, he noticed that the water in the pan was blood-stained. What, he asked his doctor, was likely to be the cause?

Blood in the pan may have come from the urine – but Paul would probably have noticed this on other occasions – or from blood coating the motions, or combined with them. Women sometimes confuse blood which has been passed from their vagina with that which has come from the bladder, rectum, or colon. Colo-rectal bleeding is often first noticed after going to the lavatory.

Bleeding from the rectum always needs an explanation, but it is surprising how long patients wait once this has happened before they consult their doctors.

The questions Paul Harrison's doctor asked him were designed to find out if the blood had originated low in the rectum, from around the anus or from higher in the colon. He wanted to know if there was bleeding at times other than when going to the lavatory. Had there been any recent change in bowel habits? Had the shape and consistency of the motions changed? Was the blood associated with pus or mucus? Was there rectal itching or pain, and, of course, was there a family history of bowel troubles – in particular, cancer?

In order to decide which part of the stomach or intestines the blood has come from, a doctor will also discuss the colour of the blood. Is it bright-red, dark cherry-red or even altered and black? Is it mixed with the stools or does the blood seem to be coating them? Is there any mucus as well as blood?

Cancers of the colon and rectum are usually slow-growing, with few symptoms in their early stages. If the tumour grows in the first part of the large colon, where the diameter of the gut is broad and the bowel's contents are still liquid, obstruction and pain are usually late symptoms, and any blood passed may well not be obvious. The patient is much more likely to notice a loss of weight, anaemia, tiredness and grumbling lower abdominal pain before blood in the motions has become apparent.

Cancer of the colon occurring nearer the rectum, where the colon is narrower and the colon walls are thicker, produces minor symptoms of partial obstruction earlier. The stools will change in diameter, they may be streaked or mixed with blood, and the pain is more likely to be colicky. Cancer of the rectum produces bright-red bleeding and the sensation that the bowels haven't been completely emptied, but pain may be absent until the tumour is well-advanced.

Many colo-rectal cancers start as benign but premalignant polyps. The chance of a polyp becoming malignant is proportional to the size it has grown. Polyps may also bleed; examination showed that, in fact, this was what was causing Paul Harrison's troubles. He will need to have regular check-ups in future in case he grows other polyps which could be premalignant.

Investigations are needed to separate the symptoms of colo-rectal cancer and colonic polyps from haemorrhoids (piles), anal fissures (small tears in the skin lining the anal canal or surrounding the anus) or some other incidental cause.

Haemorrhoids

Harry Dyson takes after his Viking ancestors. He is six feet tall, with the shoulders of a body-builder and a great beer belly. He worked all the hours God provided as a truck driver and mechanical engineer on a local farm. No load was too heavy to carry, no wheel nut too tight to loosen. Harry had, he said in a whisper that could be heard across the room, 'bleeding piles'.

Haemorrhoids, or piles, are the result of the enlargement and engorgement of the usually small vascular pads, or cushions, inside the anus. These venous patches act as draught-proofing curtains which are able to complete the closure of the anal sphincter: the muscular 'purse-string' that closes the anus.

Piles are divided into three categories. First-degree piles are invisible at the anus but they may bleed during defaecation. Second-degree haemorrhoids protrude during defaecation but then slip back afterwards spontaneously. Third-degree, or external, piles pop through the orifice and become swollen and caught, so that the patient has to push them back manually.

All three types of haemorrhoids bleed. The classic symptoms of haemorrhoids are bright-red, painless bleeding and sometimes mucus discharge. Haemorrhoids frequently cause anal irritation. Once the piles have prolapsed through the anus and become trapped beyond the anal sphincter, they may be extremely uncomfortable.

First- and second-degree haemorrhoids may well settle down with a change of diet and more regular motions. Third-degree prolapsed haemorrhoids need either injection with a sclerosing agent (an irritant solution which results in an inflammation in the veins, consequent scarring and shrinkage) or surgical treatment, whether operative or banding. The banding procedure, which is simple, involves placing a tight ring around the root of the pile so that it is starved of its blood supply and withers away.

It was always thought that piles were a penalty paid for idleness and lack of exercise, or even sitting for too long on hot radiators. It was acknowledged by traditionalists that other causes included straining because of simple constipation, or the pelvic engorgement of pregnancy coupled with pushing during delivery. Research, however, has shown that it is not the lazy weakling who is most prone to develop piles, but the strong, tough, manual worker such as Harry Dyson, who strains as he lifts sacks of cement or paving slabs.

The same patients who may suffer from piles may also develop peri-anal haematoma: small, painful clots that form in the veins found around the exterior ring of the anus. These dark-blue, pea-like lumps resolve spontaneously, but they leave behind anal skins tags – a harmless nuisance.

Harry and the thousands of people with similar troubles need careful examination. It is the oldest mistake in the book to diagnose piles without looking inside the rectum to make certain that there isn't also bleeding from a co-existent rectal cancer, or to miss some other disease of the anus or rectum.

The other trouble often confused with piles is an anal fissure. An anal fissure is a split in the skin lining the anal canal. This is not a serious condition, but it is a painful one. Fortunately, it is easily treated by medical means, or by procedures (including injections of Botox) designed to reduce the tension in the anal muscles.

IRRITABLE BOWEL SYNDROME

Fiona Robinson came into the surgery looking harassed and embarrassed. Her question, when she finally overcame her shyness and asked it, was simple. 'Doctor,' she said, 'why do I have so many attacks of diarrhoea, and why, even after I have been to the loo, do I feel that my bowel hasn't been properly emptied?'

Her unstable bowels made both her social and professional life difficult; the more important the occasion, the more quickly she had to rush from the table. Even an apparently innocuous business lunch or dinner could induce an urgent call to the loo, and to make matters worse, it could be accompanied by the even more embarrassing symptom of smelly wind. It wasn't unusual for her abdomen to become so swollen that she had to loosen the waist band of her skirt. Fiona could also be overcome by feelings of nausea and faintness while eating.

Like most of the many tens of thousands of people (mainly women) who suffer from irritable bowel syndrome (IBS), Fiona was reticent about discussing it. IBS usually starts in the twenties and thirties; it is rare for it to begin in older age groups. It is unusual for its symptoms to be troublesome once the patient has gone to sleep.

It is a nasty trick of fate that those who are naturally most sensitive are those most likely to have to bear the physically uncomfortable and socially trying symptoms of irritable bowel syndrome. IBS is the most common problem treated in the gastro-intestinal outpatients department in hospitals, and ranks with GORD (see page 72) as a reason for visiting the doctor's surgery. Irritable bowel syndrome is never diagnosed until a doctor is certain that there are no other reasons for the patient's symptoms, and that the abdominal pain or discomfort that accompanies the irregular bowel habit is relieved by defaecation.

The irregular bowel pattern may be one of intermittent diarrhoea, constipation or a mixture of both. For a diagnosis of IBS to be made, it has been decided that the symptoms must have been giving the person trouble for at least three months, and that the abnormal bowel symptoms are intermittent. The bowel movements are not accompanied by blood, but they may be associated with mucus.

Before the diagnosis is made, it is usual for the doctor to exclude other causes of bowel dysfunction, such as inflammatory bowel disease, chronic infections or cancers. Once these have been excluded, patients have to come to terms with the knowledge that there is no cure for their condition.

Even though this may sound depressing, it is often a great relief for people to know that they do not have a life-threatening condition, that now a diagnosis has been made, they are at liberty to discuss it, and that research into treatment of the problem is continuing apace. Patients should be warned that any change in the pattern of their bowel behaviour – bleeding in particular – should be reported to their doctor immediately.

The IBS patient's doctor usually makes suggestions about diet and lifestyle. Every patient is different, but most find that rich, fatty foods, too much pasta, many vegetables (especially beans and artichokes), salads (those with onions and tomatoes are particularly indigestible), and alcohol, in particular red wines and dark spirits, may trigger an attack. Coffee is also very liable to cause trouble.

Many patients find that when they are totally relaxed and eating by themselves or with their family, they can manage to eat nearly everything. However, with a new sexual partner, or at an apparently tense-free business lunch or social dinner, they can eat or drink practically nothing with impunity.

The embarrassing social difficulties that are caused by sudden diarrhoea may usually be solved by taking anti-diarrhoeal drugs such as Lomotil diphenoxylate or Imodium loperamide. Many patients find that it works better for them to take such drugs before going out to a stress-making meal rather than afterwards.

Inflammatory bowel disease

George Watts was a meticulous accountant. Neat and tidy, he was a model, if somewhat unexciting, husband and a caring father. George had the anxious, almost conspiratorial look of a patient who wants to share his worries about a problem centred below the belt. After a few comments about the present political news, he came to the point. 'Doctor, I've been feeling terrible recently. I've had a temperature. For the past few weeks I've felt ill; I have no appetite and I am losing weight. I have severe abdominal pain and I have this awful bloody diarrhoea. I am going to the lavatory five or six times a day, and I am passing large quantities of blood, and with it, pus and mucus. What's wrong? Do you think it's something I've eaten?'

Looking at George's drawn, pinched face with a flush across his cheek-bones, and his loose shirt collar – loose enough to accommodate two of my fingers – the most likely diagnosis was that he was suffering from one of the inflammatory bowel diseases (although not to be confused with irritable bowel syndrome; see page 90).

The two most common inflammatory bowel diseases are Crohn's Disease and ulcerative colitis. Although less common than IBS, these inflammatory bowel diseases are, unlike IBS, potentially serious conditions that need expert help as soon as possible. In ulcerative colitis, the ulcers erode the innermost lining (the mucosa) of the colon and rectum. Bloody diarrhoea is its hallmark.

Crohn's Disease, which is also ulcerative, usually affects the last part of the small intestine or the colon, but it may involve any part of the gastro-intestinal tract from the mouth to the anus. Unlike ulcerative colitis, it tends to erode the deeper areas of the bowel, sometimes affecting every layer of the gut wall. Whereas in ulcerative colitis the disease is essentially one of the mucosal lining of the gut, in Crohn's it affects all layers of the wall.

In ulcerative colitis, the attacks of bloody diarrhoea are usually intermittent, and there may be periods of remission. As well as the bloody diarrhoea and an urgency to go to the lavatory, the patient suffers severe cramping pain and passes quantities of mucus. Often the sufferer is ill, as George Watts was, loses weight rapidly and has a fever. The blood loss may cause anaemia, and the other symptoms lead to weight loss, an absent appetite and severe debility.

In Crohn's Disease, symptoms include chronic diarrhoea and pain, weight loss and fever. The inflamed, tender, swollen sections of gut may be felt in the lower abdomen. The gut may become obstructed by inflammation and there may be secondary malnutrition. Abscesses sometimes form around the rectum, which may also develop various fissures (splits).

If the inflammation from an inflammatory bowel disease is located near the rectum, local treatment with suppositories and enemas, usually containing steroid drugs, may ease the inflammatory processes. When, as is usually the case, the ulceration is beyond the reach of enemas, these drugs need to be taken by mouth. As well as steroids, other drugs, such as aminosalicylates, are also prescribed. For those patients who can't tolerate steroids, other immuno-suppressant drugs may be used instead.

The good news is that research is finding new methods of treating these diseases medically. When surgery is necessary and used to treat ulcerative colitis as a last resort, it often produces a dramatic improvement. Surgery may also be necessary in Crohn's Disease to remove the affected part of the gut and relieve an obstruction.

LOOK OUT FOR

Signs of Prostate Problems

having to get up at night to pass urine

being unable to last throughout a cinema
performance without a 'comfort break'

a poor urinary stream with little pressure

forked or splayed urinary stream

difficulty in starting urination

difficulty in stopping urination – 'dribbling on'

urgency – having to rush to the loo

any blood in the urine or semen

Signs of Testicular Cancer

pain in a testis

any lump in a testis

an incompletely descended
or undescended testis warrants special attention

6
MEN'S BITS
Prostate and Testicular Problems

Testicular torsion

Duncan was eighteen, rather taller and lankier than most of his contemporaries, but strong and doing well as a mechanic in the local garage. When straining to lift a heavy truck tyre, he felt a sudden pain in one of his testicles. The pain was so great that he felt sick even before he had felt his testicles and realized how tender one was. When he looked at them, he was alarmed at how one was swelling. Wisely, his foreman sent him straight round to the surgery. Was it cancer or did he have a hernia?

One look at the patient and the doctor was able to reassure Duncan. This was neither a hernia nor a cancer. It was a case of testicular torsion, which has to be treated as a surgical emergency if the testis is to be preserved.

The testicles, or testes, hang in the scrotum. This sometimes results in a twisting of the cord that supports them. The cord is accompanied by the blood supply to the testicle. Once the cord twists, the blood supply to the testicle is cut off, and gangrene will set in quickly if it is not rapidly untwisted.

Torsion of the testis is more common in young men in whom the testicles have not fully descended, or have descended late. Like all developmental problems involving the male genital tract, these often minor abnormalities are inexplicably becoming much more common. When surgeons untwist the testis affected by the torsion, they will also attach the other one more firmly so that the same thing cannot happen to it.

Sometimes, torsion of the testis may be confused with a condition that is known as epididymitis. This is an infection of the tubes that transport the sperm from the testes to the seminal vesicles, where they are stored. In epididymitis, it is usually possible to feel the thickened and tender epididymis. In young men, it almost invariably follows a urethral infection, so that a penile discharge may also be detected. The treatment for epididymitis is with the use of antibiotics.

What would have been the symptoms if Duncan had had a cancer of the testicle? If this had been the diagnosis, Duncan would have noticed, when rolling the testicle between his thumb and fingers, that one testicle had changed in shape and had a hard lump on it that removed its uniformity and made it feel different from the other. The affected testicle also often feels heavier, and the scrotum overlying it may seem swollen.

Cancers of the testis – the most common cancers to affect men from adolescence to middle age – are usually not painful. Men should regularly examine their testicles after a hot bath, when the warmth allows them to hang freely and to be readily felt.

Any changes in shape, firmness or weight, and any lump or bump should be shown to a doctor immediately – as in the case on the next page.

Testicular cancer

Philip is tall, handsome and heterosexual. When Philip was a young child, his father noticed that neither of his testes had descended into the scrotum. One could be felt in the groin, but the other was absent. Philip had surgery. One testis was removed and the other was brought down successfully into the scrotum, but it was never as firm or as large as it should have been. When Philip was twenty-four, he noticed a firm, hard lump in his remaining testicle. He asked his doctor, 'Is this cancer?'

Yes, it was. Testicular tumours are more likely to occur in men who have had maldescended testes, atrophied testes, torsion of the testes and low sperm counts, but even so, the majority of cases are found in men whose testes are otherwise absolutely normal. The death rate from the disease is higher in the professional classes than among manual workers, but no one knows why the numbers suffering from this cancer are increasing.

Like Philip, many men discover a testicular

lump only after some form of minor trauma, but evidence suggests that this merely draws attention to the testes. Testicular cancer may be painless or painful. The only safe rule is to show any testicular lump to the doctor so that he can examine it and, if necessary, arrange for a painless ultrasound examination of it.

All men should examine their testes as carefully and as regularly as women examine their breasts. The testis is examined by rolling it between the finger and thumb after a hot bath while the man is standing up. Any absent testicle lurking in the abdomen should be removed; those brought down into the scrotum should be examined routinely even more carefully. Similarly, once a patient has suffered a torsion of the testis, both testes should be observed and felt regularly.

Philip was treated and, like over ninety-five percent of men who now have cancer of the testis, he has had no further trouble.

STRANGULATED PENIS

Simon Davies is twenty-three and a bit of a lad. At home with his girlfriend one evening, he was just about to make love to her when his foreskin, which had been drawn back, became tight. This restricted the circulation to the penis, so that it became grossly swollen and very painful. Simon rang his doctor at once. 'Something terrible has happened to my penis,' he said. 'It has been strangled by my foreskin. Can you help?'

Doctors used to reducing paraphimoses ('strangulated penises') can usually restore normality by gentle but firm manipulation, sometimes after an injection to reduce the swelling, or the use of ice. Simon's anxiety and misery were rapidly relieved. If manipulation fails, a general anaesthetic may be needed. Occasionally, a doctor may need to perform an immediate circumcision. In any event, Simon would be advised to have a circumcision so that it doesn't occur again. The basic cause is too small an opening to the foreskin.

PROSTATE GLAND ENLARGEMENT

Henry was sixty-three. Usually neat, tidy and alert, he looked depressed, and there was an unmistakable whiff of urine when he came into the surgery. It was possible to guess what his question would be about before it was asked. 'Doctor,' he said gloomily, 'I don't know what has happened to my waterworks. I can't stop leaking. What's causing this?'

A few questions revealed that Henry had all the classic signs of prostatic enlargement. The overwhelming majority of people who experience prostatic enlargement have a benign enlargement of the prostate gland, also known as benign prostatic hyperplasia, or BPH.

In those cases in which the prostate is malignant and so big that it causes symptoms similar to those about which Henry was complaining, treatment may be possible, but it is probably already too late for a cure. Conversely, benign prostatic enlargement is readily treated, either surgically or medically.

Only if it is neglected is the patient likely to suffer long-term problems.

As Henry had already discovered, although BPH is described as benign because it is not cancerous, its symptoms can cause social as well as medical problems.

Life is difficult enough without having to face it after a broken night's sleep. His lacklustre appearance was the result of sleeplessness. Many ageing men with enlarged prostates have to get up to pass urine several times a night, with the result that both their sleep, and their partners', is fragmented.

Difficulties in passing urine because of the enlargement of the prostate result in the bladder being incompletely emptied, and the residual pool of urine left in the bladder may readily become infected. As the obstruction from the enlarging prostate progressively blocks the urethra (the tube that leads from the bladder through the penis and to the outside world), the urinary stream becomes increasingly feeble. There is 'dribbling on' after peeing (known as post-micturition dribble) so that the finest pair of trousers may be ruined, and the patient may, like Henry, start to smell.

Patients may also notice that the urinary stream is no longer a single jet but may be splayed or forked, so that bathroom carpets become sodden. As patients with an enlarging prostate have to pass urine so often, they can no longer sit throughout a complete cinema performance or a restaurant meal without having to take a break. They may also have urgency of micturition – a medical term meaning that they have to rush to the lavatory lest they be caught short.

All these symptoms have occurred because, as men grow older, their prostate gland enlarges, and, because the prostate surrounds the urethra and the more it grows, the tighter it grips the urethra until it becomes increasingly difficult to pass water. Henry is in plentiful company. Over a third of men at fifty and more than half those aged sixty have some enlargement of the prostate, and by the age of eighty-five, nine out of ten have benign prostatic hyperplasia. In about half the cases in which the prostate has become enlarged, active treatment, either medical or surgical, is needed.

When blood tests, including a simple PSA (prostatic specific antigen blood test; see page 110), showed that Henry didn't have cancer, he opted to have surgery: a trans-urethral re-section of the prostate, known as a TURP, which remains the gold standard for treatment.

Although this is now a routine procedure, it has one common disadvantage. Following surgery, the majority of patients experience something called retrograde ejaculation; when this happens, the semen during ejaculation flows back into the bladder. Men complain that this causes some loss of quality in their sex lives. Medical treatment has now so improved that it is an acceptable first-response treatment for BPH.

PROSTATE CANCER

David was much the same age as Henry. He looked very well when he came to the surgery for a chat about his gout. He was the chief executive of a prosperous provincial company and was happily married, but even so, he had the reputation of being a bit of a womanizer. He enjoyed all the good things of life, including wine and rich foods.

Having exhausted everything that could be said about David's gout, the doctor asked him a question. 'David, have you had your PSA done?' David looked surprised and replied, 'No. What's a PSA?' David is among the majority of men who don't know about PSA, the potentially life-saving prostatic specific antigen blood test which is a better diagnostic test than either mammography or cervical screening – both of which are so well-known to women.

If cancer of the prostate is to be treated at a time and stage in its development when a cure is still possible, it may be – probably *will* be –

fatal to wait until the prostate is so big that it is obstructing the flow of urine or is causing bleeding into the urine or semen.

Fortunately, cancer of the prostate can now be detected when it is not producing any symptoms. At this stage, the chance of a cure is still possible with a great majority of cases, provided the nature of the cancer cells doesn't make the cancer unusually malignant. Silent, malignantly enlarged prostates can be detected via the PSA test.

PSA is an enzyme that is produced in the prostate gland. It only passes into the bloodstream in unusually large quantities when the prostate cells are damaged by malignancy or infection.

When the doctor discovers that there is more than usual PSA in the blood, more detailed examinations may then be organized. These may include a trans-rectal ultrasound, in which the prostate gland is scanned by an ultrasound placed in the rectum. Although this sounds unpleasant, it is no more than uncomfortable and not painful.

A biopsy of the prostate is usually taken at

the same time as the rectal ultrasound. The specimens are preferably collected from those areas the ultrasound has shown to be suspicious. The discomfort caused by the biopsy varies from patient to patient; it probably depends on the readiness with which the patient bleeds and the size of the gland. Even in those unusual cases in which the procedure is painful, the pain rapidly wears off. Most patients think it is a small price to pay either for an early diagnosis and the chance of a normal life span, or simply for the reassurance it provides.

Another method of detecting cancer of the prostate is with a digital examination of the gland – that is, via the rectum with the doctor's finger. Even the most experienced doctor is only able to detect malignant changes when they can be felt on the posterior aspects of the prostate. Even so, this can be invaluable in detecting tumours in some of the minority of patients who have prostate cancer, yet in whom the PSA is not raised.

There is some controversy about the regular screening of male patients for prostatic cancer.

Although this may be the only way to detect the disease when it can still be cured, some doctors feel that the anxiety it may cause some patients and the expense of ultrasound and biopsy do not justify its widespread use in an aged population with an inevitably limited life span.

This is not my view. In my opinion, men should know their PSA level once they are fifty – forty if there is a family history – and the test should ideally be repeated annually. Improvements in radiotherapy and in hormone therapy mean that most men with cancer of the prostate, however old, will have a longer, more active life, and will benefit from early diagnosis, provided they are given adequate treatment.

LOOK OUT FOR

Signs of Breast Cancer

any breast lump

discharge or bleeding from the nipple

scaly rash around the nipple

dimpling of the breast skin

any change in shape of the breast

swollen glands in the armpits

pain in the breast

7

WOMEN'S BITS
Breast and Ovarian Problems

Benign breast lumps

Angela is in her early forties. Her successful business career has been interrupted just once: when she had her only child. She is tall, thin, well-exercised and efficient, and she usually plays as hard as she works. One night when having a bath, she discovered a lump in her still-firm breast. Next morning, she was at her doctor's. Controlled but tense, her question was direct. 'What is this lump? Can you be sure it isn't cancer?'

The doctor examined Angela's breasts and was able to give her some reassurance immediately. He said that eighty-five percent of all breast lumps found by a patient and brought to the doctor's attention prove to be non-malignant. Even so, as investigating them could prove to be life-saving, it was never a waste of time.

An important factor (and arguably *the* most important) that determines survival in breast cancer is early diagnosis. If the breast lump is less than an inch in diameter and has not spread, the woman has a ninety-five percent chance of long-term survival.

The doctor went on to explain to Angela that breasts could be compared to pillows. Three out of four breasts were similar to the best-quality pillows: soft, uniform and free of lumps and bumps. However, one in four breasts are lumpy, bumpy and nodular, and feel more like the type of pillow found in a third-rate hotel.

Angela had nodular breasts, and the lump she had found was a nodule that was bigger than the rest. Benign lumps found in breasts are usually either the result of fibrocystic disease of the breast (referred to by many patients as 'lumpy, bumpy' breasts) or fibro-adenomas. Both conditions are benign.

Fibrocystic disease is most commonly found in premenopausal women. They often notice that their breasts are slightly painful and tender before a period and that they may well vary in size according to the stage in the cycle. There is debate as to whether malignancy is more common in fibrocystic disease, but there is agreement that if a malignant tumour does occur in a fibrocystic breast, it is more easily missed. The presence of benign lumps, whether from adenomata or fibrocystic disease, certainly doesn't protect against cancer.

A fibroadenoma tends to be found as a single painless lump that is freely moveable in the breast tissue and has the consistency of India rubber. These can occur in any age group, but are more common in younger women in their twenties and thirties. Even though they are benign, they need removing by an excision biopsy, so that everyone may rest assured that an error hasn't been made in diagnosis. Fibroadenoma of the breast may be recurrent.

Angela, as the doctor who had treated her for years would have expected, knew the make-up of her breasts well, and had behaved wisely by seeking expert help at once. There is discussion about the usefulness of women formally feeling their breasts, in the same way as doctors do, at regular intervals at the same time of the cycle. This used to be considered a very useful procedure, but recently it has been suggested that what is important is not so much the formal monthly examination, but a woman's awareness of the make-up of her own breasts and the immediate recognition when they feel different.

Like many women with fibrocystic breasts, Angela had had some breast pain at period times. She was, however, aware that breast pain is a totally unreliable symptom when diagnosing breast lumps. There is not a doctor practising who hasn't had a patient who was misled into thinking that a benign tumour was malignant because it was painful, or a cancer was benign because it had no pain – and vice versa in both cases. As these mistakes can have tragic consequences, women should disregard the diagnostic relevance of pain and show all breast lumps to their doctor.

Angela was referred for ultrasound and fine-needle aspiration: the use of a narrow-bored needle to draw some fluid from the breast nodule so that the cells can be examined. The results of both procedures were negative.

BREAST CANCER

The doctor knew Monica well. A surgery regular, she was sixty-five and overweight, with large breasts. Monica was over-fond of good rich food, under-exercised, and drank rather more than usual. Her periods had continued long after fifty-two – the average age of the menopause – until she was fifty-six. She had had only one child, which she hadn't breast-fed. Her grandmother and one aunt had had cancer of the breast. Monica hadn't had regular mammographies, so she wanted the doctor to examine her breasts in case this had resulted in an undiscovered tumour. Did he, she asked, think this was possible?

Even as Monica was talking, the doctor was ticking off a mental list of the various risk factors that make breast cancer more likely. Most breast cancers have a hormonal link, so that anything which increases oestrogen levels in the body increases the likelihood of breast cancer. Breast cancer occurs more often in women who start their periods before their contemporaries and stop them (have the menopause) later than normal.

Women who have used a high-dose contraceptive pill; those who have used oestrogen-based contraceptive pills under the age of twenty-one or after thirty-six; women who have used HRT and, in particular, have continued with it beyond the age of fifty-eight; and those who are overweight or have had a rich western diet or regular alcohol (both of which increase oestrogen levels) all have a fractionally increased risk of breast cancer – albeit lifestyle and diet may confer other health benefits.

Conversely, breast cancer risk is decreased by pregnancies and breast-feeding. A strong family history is found in some cases of breast cancer. Although breast cancer may be common in those people with these characteristics, the great majority of cases are found in patients who don't have any so-called risk factor.

Any distinct lump in the breast should have a doctor's opinion. A breast cancer feels firm, sometimes even hard. It may become associated with other signs of breast trouble if the lump hasn't been found when still very small.

When small, the cancer isn't usually attached to either the skin or the underlying muscle and can be moved easily in the surrounding breast tissue. Once the tumour has become better established, it becomes attached to the overlying skin, which may become dimpled like that of orange peel; as a result and in time, the contours and size of the breast are altered. A more advanced cancer also becomes tied down to the chest muscles.

Some breast cancers are associated with a nipple discharge or bleeding, symptoms that always needs investigation, although only a minority of nipple discharges are malignant. With some cancers, the nipple becomes obviously indrawn (inverted). One type of breast malignancy may make itself known by the presence of an eczema-type rash on the nipple. If a gland under the arm is firm and swollen, suspicions are aroused.

A mammogram confirmed the doctor's fears. Monica did indeed have a breast cancer, but fortunately, although she had taken risks by not having regular mammography, it was still at a very early stage. The pathologists reported that the cells in the cancer were not unusually malignant and that the tumour cells had hormone receptors, which showed that they would be sensitive to tamoxifen or one of the other recently introduced oestrogen-blocking drugs.

The omens were excellent. A lumpectomy (local surgery), radiotherapy and tamoxifen (or similar drug) should mean that there is every likelihood that Monica would achieve her expected life span of eighty-three. She promised to have mammography in future.

Ovarian tumours

Mrs Mackintosh, aged sixty, had read that the most common time of life to develop ovarian cancer was between the ages of fifty and seventy, and that it was more prevalent in industrialized societies. She had also learned that the most frequent symptoms of ovarian cancer were indigestion and bloating, an inability to enjoy a large meal (satiety), wind, constipation, a urinary leak and backache. Mrs Mackintosh worried that she might be one of the middle-aged women who suffer from this, the most common cancers of the female genital organs (the standard textbook lists twenty different types) – more common, even, than cancer of the cervix and body of the womb combined. Her question was therefore simple: 'How do you know that I haven't got cancer of the ovaries?'

The truthful answer is that diagnosing cancer of the ovary is very difficult in the absence of other symptoms. Consequently, two-thirds of cases are only diagnosed at a late stage.

Treatment is still possible, but the longer it has been present, the less likely the chances of a cure.

The symptoms that Mrs Macintosh had read about are all symptoms of advanced cancer. Early cancer of the ovary has no symptoms; when it is diagnosed at an early stage, it is because it has usually been discovered by chance while other procedures are being carried out.

Ovarian cancer is more common if there is a strong family history of ovarian, breast or colon cancer. Even so, fewer than five percent of cases of ovarian cancer can be definitely related to what are called the BRCA genes, which are known to have a strong association with it.

Ovarian cancer is also more common in those women who have not had children, or who had them late, and if they haven't taken the contraceptive pill for a long portion of their reproductive lives. Taking the pill – or later, HRT – reduces the likelihood of developing ovarian cancer, whereas a late menopause favours a diagnosis of ovarian cancer. The search is on to find a better and more reliable marker for cancer of the ovary. In the meantime, the marker CA 125 may give valuable clues in some cases.

Patients who are concerned about ovarian cancer usually have a vaginal examination. By the time they are Mrs Mackintosh's age, the ovaries are usually small, so that any lumps and bumps in the ovarian area merit careful examination and a blood test.

Ordinary trans-abdominal ultrasound is a poor way of detecting ovarian cancer, and the preferred method is to use transvaginal ultrasound with a sonograph placed in the vagina. In skilled hands, this can prove a very useful diagnostic tool, as it differentiates between cysts and tumours, but to be certain of the diagnosis, biopsy is necessary.

All Mrs Mackintosh's tests were negative. It was wise to check out any worries, and the doctor reassured her that her symptoms – the swelling abdomen, bloating, change in weight, indigestion, constipation and incontinence – were all far more likely to be caused by conditions other than cancer of the ovary – albeit they may merit further investigation.

Mrs Mackintosh's vague symptoms were the reason why she quite rightly sought her doctor's advice. Luckily he was able to reassure her that, worrying as these symptoms can occasionally be, she had nothing to be concerned about. Other women are faced with a similar but different problem after abdominal surgery.

If a woman needs to have her abdomen opened up after the menopause, when the ovaries cease to function but may still undergo malignant change, many doctors suggest that she should have the ovaries removed while the surgeon is in a position to do so. This question is particularly likely to be asked if the patient has a hysterectomy; it is only a matter of moments to extend the operation by removing the ovaries as well. Similarly, a simple operation like the removal of an appendix is not rendered more complex by removing the ovaries. Even though the ovaries are shrivelled and no longer produce hormones, they remain a potential source of cancer from which one woman in seventy at some time in her life is destined to suffer.

LOOK OUT FOR

Signs of Sexual Problems

In men

discharge from the penis or anus

meatal lips (the penile opening)
stuck together in the morning

pain on passing urine

pain in the testis

sores, ulcers, warts, skin tags in the
genital or perianal area

In women

discharge

pain on passing urine

lower abdominal pain

sores, ulcers, warts, skin tags

irregular bleeding, bleeding after intercourse,
post-menopausal bleeding, bleeding when pregnant

8
TROUBLE DOWN BELOW
Sexual Problems & Vaginal Bleeding

Painful intercourse

It took Mrs Rendle, who is forty-five, some weeks to pluck up the courage to go and see her doctor. After a chat about her back and the doctor's garden, she finally came to the point. 'I've been having very painful intercourse for the past few months,' she explained. 'I wonder what can be wrong?'

Pain on intercourse – known technically as dyspareunia – is divided into two types: deep dyspareunia and superficial dyspareunia. Mrs Rendle's pain was felt when her husband first penetrated her; this type of pain is classified as superficial dyspareunia.

Superficial dyspareunia is very common; rarely a day goes by without a GP being asked about it. The most frequent cause is lack of lubrication. Women are well aware that when they become sexually aroused, even interested, there is an increased production of the lubricating fluid in the vagina and from the glands at the entrance of the vagina. If a woman is tired, has reduced sexual desire for any reason, or sometimes even when she is constipated, less lubrication than usual is produced.

The production of the lubricant is associated with some swelling from engorgement of the female external genitalia, including the clitoris and vulva. This is the equivalent of an erection in a man. Alcohol may also reduce lubrication: the female equivalent of 'brewer's droop'. Women who are in Mrs Rendle's age group – approaching the menopause – may well notice that they produce less lubrication than they did and have less engorgement, even if their libido is unaltered or, in some cases, increased.

In their later years, women's desire may increase, even if their ability to act on it may decrease. The latter is the result of lower oestrogen levels, whereas an increase in libido may be due to a proportional increase in testosterone levels (women have it, too). Blood tests will show whether the menopause is approaching and whether either HRT or KY jelly could be an answer to the problem.

Other causes of superficial pain on intercourse include thrush, herpes, atrophic vaginitis (the narrowing and thinning of the vagina after the menopause) or other incidental infections or injuries. The discharge of thrush and other infections, however profuse, is a poor lubricant and it may cause painful intercourse, however strong the desire.

Deep dyspareunia is pain felt in the pelvis and low in the abdomen once intercourse has started. It is a different type of pain from that of superficial dyspareunia. The abdominal tenderness may be so severe as to induce nausea, and it is brought on or made worse by movement of the female abdominal organs – ovaries, tubes and uterus – which results from a man's thrusting during intercourse.

Deep dyspareunia should always have a gynaecological opinion. Among its many causes are ovarian problems, fibroids and frequently pelvic inflammatory disease (often the result of chlamydial infection).

Vaginismus is an occasional cause of painful intercourse. Trouble occurs once intercourse begins, usually when the woman is first touched genitally, but if not, then when penetration is attempted. The vagina reacts by going into a painful spasm. This is one problem that is psychological in nature, but if the patient, her partner and her medical advisors all persevere, it almost invariably responds to psychotherapy.

Sexual infections

George Ellis was a regular at the genito-urinary medical clinic (or GUM, previously known as a special or VD clinic). His question was uncomplicated. 'What do you think the discharge is this time doctor? I think it's NSU.'

Although George was a regular visitor to his local GUM, these clinics are attended by an almost equal number of men and women from all walks of life. The doctors and nurses in the clinics pride themselves on their easy-going, non-judgmental approach to life and medicine. Although busy, and very much busier than they used to be, they are still prepared to discuss any trouble or worry about the health, anatomy and physiology of those parts found between the belly button and the thigh – what patients often refer to as 'down there'.

Despite gender differences, the signs and symptoms of sexual infections are comparable in both sexes. George had noticed pain on passing urine. He described it as sharp and burning. He thought that the tip of his penis was slightly redder than usual, and had observed that when he passed water for the first time in the morning, the lips of his penis were crusty and stuck together. He now had a slight pale-cream but watery discharge.

He was right: he had non-specific urethritis, or NSU, which is usually, but not always, the result of a chlamydial urethritis. George was treated by an appropriate course of antibiotics. In addition, Myra and Susanne, his two girlfriends, and their partners were seen and treated.

Chlamydial infections in women are often more insidious than in men. A slight urethral discharge in an already moist area that is hidden by the vulval lips is easily missed. The minimal pain or discomfort of urethritis is too easily dismissed by a woman as being nothing more than a mild attack of cystitis. Others may attribute it to not drinking enough, so that their urine has become too concentrated.

Unfortunately, while they are all too readily disregarded, chlamydial infections are of great importance to women as they are the most common cause of pelvic inflammatory disease and the most frequent reason for their tubes becoming blocked and for natural pregnancy becoming impossible. Any woman whose partner has NSU must also be treated. Pain or discomfort on passing water, when coupled with low abdominal pain, always needs investigation to exclude chlamydia.

Gonorrhoea has signs and symptoms that are similar to those produced by chlamydial infections, but the gonococcal bacteria usually produce (with occasional exceptions) a much more profuse and darker yellow discharge, together with greater pain on passing urine. In men, a discharge is often so heavy that it soaks through their clothing – meaning that it is difficult to ignore.

The other most common infections people acquire sexually include trichonomas vaginalis, or TV, which gives rise to a frothy, white, very irritating discharge in women, but usually no more than a minuscule clear discharge (and sometimes not even that) in men.

Venereal or genital warts are fleshy and unsightly. They occur around the genitalia and perianal region. Unattractive as they are, the more obvious genital warts are not the dangerous ones, but they may serve as markers for the almost-invisible warts which are caused by the human papilloma virus, or HPV. In a few cases, infection with HPV may lead later to cancer of the cervix, and, less often, probably of the penis and anus.

Herpes is well-known. Everyone has seen cold sores around the mouth which are caused by the oral herpes virus, herpes Type 1. Genital herpes – herpes Type 2 – is the counterpart 'down below'. Both types may flourish at either site. In severe or recurrent cases, herpes can be treated or kept at bay by taking an antiviral agent such as Zovirax aciclovir or Valtrex valaciclovir.

Vaginal bleeding

Susie Brown is a thirty-four-year-old teacher. She is married and has no children, despite having been 'trying' for over a year. On the way home after school, she noticed that, although it wasn't time for her period, she had some vaginal bleeding. Rather than going home for tea, she turned round and went to the doctor's surgery.

Being wise and fearful of making a serious mistake, the doctor immediately remembered an old adage that any woman who has missed a period or who complains of vaginal bleeding between the ages of fifteen and fifty is pregnant unless there is evidence to the contrary. The two possibilities that sprang immediately to the doctor's mind were that Susie could be pregnant and that she might either be threatening to miscarry, actually starting to miscarry, or – more alarmingly – that the bleeding could be the first sign of an ectopic pregnancy.

An ectopic pregnancy is the condition in

which a fertilized ovum has implanted and is growing in the fallopian tube rather than in the uterus. Ectopic pregnancies are more likely to be experienced by a woman who has had difficulty in conceiving, as in many instances the infertility is the result of fallopian tubes having been damaged by past infection – a similar origin to that of ectopic pregnancies. The stage of pregnancy at which problems start in an ectopic pregnancy depends on where the egg has become implanted, but it is usually between the eighth and twelfth week.

The doctor's first questions were designed to find out if Susie had missed a period, and if her last period was normal in every respect. She asked about any breast activity or morning sickness and whether Susie had noticed that her tummy appeared swollen. The abdominal muscles become lax in very early pregnancy, and as a result, the tummy sticks out long before it is pushed out by the growth of the baby.

Susie had missed a period. The urine tests the doctor did in the surgery confirmed that she was pregnant. Fortunately, in this case there was no evidence of an ectopic pregnancy or that the threatened miscarriage had become an inevitable miscarriage; the cervix was still closed. Susie continued with her pregnancy and had a normal baby at term.

Ectopic pregnancies are always much more dangerous for women than miscarriages. With a ruptured ectopic pregnancy, there is usually severe abdominal pain and an acutely tender lower abdomen with, on vaginal examination, extreme tenderness over the affected tube. There may be gross bleeding internally, even if the bleeding from the vagina is comparatively light. The woman may be shocked: sweating, pale, collapsed, with a quick, feeble pulse and a blood pressure that is barely detectable. A ruptured ectopic is a medical emergency.

Late in pregnancy, any bleeding may signal an emergency and needs to be reported to the doctor immediately. This bleeding usually stems from the detachment of part of the placenta, whether because it is unfortunately attached over the internal opening of the neck of the womb (cervix), or a damaged placenta as the result of raised blood pressure or some incidental cause. Whatever the cause, it needs immediate medical attention.

Irregular vaginal bleeding (at an unexpected time) and in the absence of pregnancy, or bleeding (even spotting) after intercourse always needs early investigation. It could be related to troubles with the womb, disease of the cervix, an infection in the vagina or atrophic vaginitis: the post-menopausal thinning of the vagina. Post-menopausal bleeding should be investigated as soon as possible. Very occasionally, bleeding occurs from the vagina as the result of some blood-clotting disorder.

WILLY WORRIES

Dennis was eighteen. His doctor had known him since he was a small child, so that when he came into the surgery and fidgeted wildly as he sat on his chair, he guessed the question would concern sex. The majority of patients who consult their doctor about a sexual problem don't have a sexual disease but have noticed some perfectly normal variation in their genitalia or have some anxiety. Dennis was no exception. After a few embarrassed comments about Chelsea's recent performance, he came out with it: 'Doctor, my penis is too small. Can I have it enlarged?'

Even a doctor who has spent half a lifetime working in a genito-urinary clinic finds it difficult to reassure men suffering from this particular anxiety – increasingly referred to as 'willy worries'. Even so, some good is done by explaining to men, whatever their age, that other men's penises are usually nothing like as large or as active as their bragging owners claim.

When erect and measured along its upper

length, the average penis is somewhere between four-and-a-half to seven inches long – more than enough to cope with the average length of a woman's vagina, which measures approximately three to four inches. Seven to eight inches is a large penis, and a nine-inch penis strikes dread even into the most hardened East End prostitute. When I worked in a Whitechapel clinic, the local prostitutes, who at that time used to trade from Brick Lane, would spy any regular punter who boasted a nine-inch organ as soon as he came into the street and then draw lots to decide who should cope with him.

Contrary to the popular belief reinforced by agony aunts, size *does* matter, but moderation in everything is what really counts. Research in the early nineties showed that although fifteen percent of men thought women admired a large penis, only two percent of women were interested in what it looked like. Questioning prostitutes, who have little, if any, emotional interest in their clients but in many cases are sexually responsive, the preference is for an average-sized male organ of slightly above-average girth – as one said to me, 'a cigar rather than a cigarette'.

While nothing to do with Dennis's concerns, The other two most frequent worries men share with their doctors concern impotency and premature ejaculation.

It is not always much help telling a man that premature ejaculation stems either from excessive enthusiasm (overwhelming desire) or from anxiety and tension. Masters and Johnson-type exercises, in which the man becomes gradually accustomed to shared intimacy and lovemaking so that he becomes increasingly relaxed with his partner, are helpful but time-consuming.

Other patients may prefer to try one of the class of drugs known as 5HT re-uptake inhibitors, in particular Seroxat paroxetine. A small dose may delay orgasm and ejaculation if taken when needed. These drugs were introduced for the treatment of depression, but it was soon found that some of them had a side-effect on sexual response. The effect was variable, but enough men benefited for its fame to spread, and the queue at my clinic began to snake through the hospital waiting room and into the street.

Viagra has revolutionized the treatment of impotence. Impotence was once thought of as being mainly a psychological problem. Now it is known that between seventy and eighty percent of cases are solely the consequence of a physical problem; in many other cases there may be a mixed pattern. In many instances a man's confidence is so eroded by a weakening response as the result of failing prowess that he begins to fear intercourse. Once confidence is restored, potency recovers.

Viagra and similar drugs are only successful when some sexual desire is present; they do not restore an absent libido. In cases where there is surgical or traumatic destruction of the nerves leading to the pelvis, Viagra is of little benefit.

LOOK OUT FOR

Early Signs of Diabetes

weight loss despite eating well

increased frequency of urination

increased thirst • loss of energy

tiredness • blurred vision

infections which heal slowly • thrush

Early Signs of Over-Active Thyroid

weight loss • palpitations

heat intolerance • agitation

irritability • sleeplessness

over-active bowels

Early Signs of Under-Active Thyroid

slow pulse • hoarse voice

dry skin and lacklustre hair

tiredness • loss of emotion

constipation

9

DODGY HORMONES
Diabetes and Thyroid Diseases

DIABETES

Charlotte Winstanley is a fifty-year-old house-wife. She works three days a week supervising children's school meals. Whatever spare time Charlotte has left over from looking after her family of four and the school work, she devotes to the church. Charlotte never rests. Overweight and too busy to take much exercise, Charlotte was eventually forced to see the doctor because she was feeling tired and generally unwell. She had also noticed that she had been unusually hungry over the past few months. Her symptoms were so vague that all she could say to the doctor was, 'Where has all my energy gone?'

The doctor realized that Mrs Winstanley wouldn't have taken time off unless something significant was amiss. His first thought on seeing her was that she had lost weight, and he immediately began to wonder whether she might have some hidden cancer, although this seemed unlikely as her appetite had increased.

Questioning revealed that Mrs Winstanley had noticed an ever-decreasing loss of energy so that her over-crowded programme was becoming more and more difficult to maintain. She hadn't previously realized that she had lost weight, but after consideration agreed that her clothes were much looser. She denied that there was any loss of appetite and said that, if anything, she was more hungry than usual.

When asked about her waterworks, Charlotte said that she was getting up several times during the night to pass urine, and also passing it more frequently by day. She thought this constant loo-visiting had produced inflammation and irritation around her genitalia and groin.

The doctor continued with his routine questions, but once he had heard that Mrs Winstanley was losing weight (despite eating more and being increasingly hungry), was thirsty, urinating more frequently and feeling lacklustre and short of energy, he knew he had the diagnosis: diabetes mellitus. Further questioning showed that recently Charlotte's eyesight was becoming a bit blurred. She also explained that, a month of two ago, she had suffered a boil on her neck which had taken a long while to heal.

The symptoms of diabetes are weight loss (often combined with an increased appetite); frequency of urination; in both sexes, thrush around the genitalia and in other moist parts of the body, therefore soreness and irritation; reduced resistance to skin infections; loss of energy; and sometimes tingling or burning sensations in the hands or feet.

Mrs Winstanley has Type 2 diabetes. This affects two million people in the UK and used to be known as non-insulin-dependent diabetes or late-onset diabetes. It develops slowly, usually (but by no means always) in middle-aged and older people who are frequently overweight and don't get enough exercise.

Conversely, Type 1 diabetes, an acute disease, develops mainly in younger people (adolescents, young adults, sometimes children) who are often previously thin and athletic. The same symptoms but more acute and more severe occur as in Type 2 diabetes. They may be associated with vomiting, stomach pain, sweating, some loss of vision and headaches, and if not treated promptly, confusion and loss of consciousness. The start of Type 1 diabetes may create a medical emergency.

Early treatment of Type 2 diabetes is also essential if serious and permanent damage to the eyes, kidneys, heart and the arteries leading to the feet (and hence gangrene) is to be prevented. When the diagnosis is being made, blood tests are taken to determine the patient's present blood sugar and the average blood sugar for the past two months. Diagnosis is confirmed by carefully timed blood tests taken after eating. Urine-testing is a rough check, but not as efficient as blood tests, particularly in elderly patients.

Patients taking insulin, or occasionally oral medication, may have hypoglycaemic attacks (low blood sugar). Irritability, sweating, slurred speech, tremulousness may give way to blurred vision, confusion and coma. The immediate treatment is glucose, whether as sugar, sweets, sweet drinks and later a meal.

Thyroid problems

Mary Eardley is a forty-one-year-old research assistant. Her job is as stressful as her boss is difficult. When Mary noticed that she was sweating more than usual so that her palms were hot and sticky, was losing weight despite a good appetite, and was becoming so irritable that she was losing her temper with her employer (who was no worse than usual), she grew concerned. She thought that all she needed was a good holiday away from the office – in particular, from the telephone, which enraged her every time it rang.

Yet when she returned from a fortnight in Morocco, Mary was no better. In fact, she had become aware of other troubling symptoms. She had found heat intolerable, although on a visit to the Nile the previous year she had been able to walk to the tombs without noticing it. Her bowels had been much more active, although she hadn't succumbed to the local bugs. On a walking tour into the hills, she hadn't been able to keep up: her heart had raced, she had had palpitations and felt weak.

As soon as she returned home, Mary went to see her doctor, had a row with the receptionist about being kept waiting, and then presented him with a neatly drawn up list of her troubles. 'Doctor,' she said, 'every part of me seems to be in trouble. What is the matter with me?'

The doctor already had his answer. He had seen Mary on his way through the waiting room and had noticed that she was agitated, aggressive, had lost weight and that her eyes were slightly more prominent (and glistening); the whites could even be seen around the iris. When she made her hectic way to her chair in the consulting room, he remembered an old adage: if a doctor doesn't diagnose an over-active thyroid the moment he sees a patient with hyperthyroidism, he will starve.

Sure enough, as soon as Mary held out her hands for the doctor, her fingers showed a fine shake (tremor). Holding her chin still with one hand, the doctor asked her to look up at a finger of his other hand, which he held above her head, and to follow it down as he lowered it. He saw that Mary's eyeballs came down faster than the eyelids, so that there was a fraction of a moment when a large expanse of the white of her eye showed above her dark-brown iris. Her reflexes were brisker than usual.

The doctor then went through her list of symptoms. He explained that every tissue and organ in the body needed the correct quantity of thyroid hormones, and that this was why Mary had complained that no part of her seemed to be working the way it used to.

Mary was told that it was important to have her thyroid treated, for while her boss may not have worried about her increased aggressiveness, others would be upset by her rages. Above all, she needed urgent treatment, because running her heart at this rate could demand more from it than it could provide. This could lead to atrial fibrillation (see page 38) or it could even precipitate heart failure.

Once her over-active thyroid had been regulated with the use of carbimazole and, for a short time, beta blockers, a close check was kept on Mary's thyroid activity so that if she relapsed, surgery or radiotherapy with radioactive iodine could be used. So far, Mary hasn't needed any further medical treatment.

The opposite thyroid problem, hypothyroidism (too little thyroid hormone), is often misdiagnosed. Between three and four percent of people over the age of sixty-five unknowingly suffer from it, and not all symptoms are present or marked. Patients may become excessively unemotional and dull, with a hoarse voice and a slowness of speech. They are constipated, suffer from the cold, have a slow pulse and put on weight. Their hair becomes coarse and dry, and their skin is parchment-like and scaly. They may be affected by a raised cholesterol level.

Whenever an older person starts to become unusually lethargic or someone of any age has a raised cholesterol level, a simple blood test should be done to make sure the thyroid gland is working effectively.

LOOK OUT FOR

Recurring Urinary Tract Infections

blood in the urine

cystitis which rapidly recurs or
doesn't respond to antibiotics

pain on passing urine

frequency of passing urine

pain in loins
(the part of the back over the kidneys)

these could all be signs of disease which need
immediate investigation

10
WATERWORKS
Urinary Diseases

Urinary tract infections

Peter Johnson, a fifty-five-year-old lawyer who was overweight, under-exercised, overfed and a heavy social drinker, was always a welcome patient on the few occasions when he visited the surgery. Amiable and easy-going, he took an interest in his problems (when he had any), cooperated with his treatment and was invariably polite to other patients and staff. All these qualities were going to be put to the test when he came to ask the doctor about his urine. 'Doctor,' he said, 'there's just the pinkest tinge to my urine. Do you think it's blood?'

The list of different causes for blood in the urine, or haematuria, is a long one, and they vary from the alarming to the trivial. Often, the investigations for assessing blood in the urine are tiresome and intimate, and ultimately don't reveal any serious cause. However, not to investigate them thoroughly and immediately could sometimes be depriving the patient of a cure for a potentially fatal condition.

The important message, understood by

doctors but not always by patients, is that however little the blood – even if it is microscopic and can only be detected either in the laboratory or by the use of one of the special dipsticks used to check urine in the surgery – it still needs urgent investigation. Research has shown that blood in the urine is still a symptom that is underrated by the general public. The result is that too many patients' lives are put in danger by late diagnosis.

The most common cause of blood in the urine is urethritis or cystitis (an infection in the urethra or bladder, respectively), or an infection in the upper urinary tract, the kidney or the collecting system (the renal pelvis) leading to the ureter and from there to the bladder. Infection in this part of the urinary tract is known as pyelonephritis. This is associated with all the usual symptoms of cystitis – frequency of urination, urgency, pain on passing urine, fever and lower abdominal pain – together with pain and tenderness in the renal angle between the lower ribs and the spine. People with pyelonephritis frequently have a very high temperature accompanied by shivering attacks (rigors).

Even if there is no bleeding, cystitis that recurs often or doesn't respond in the expected way to treatment also needs thorough investigation, as it may be a sign of an underlying disease of the bladder, including a malignancy.

In men of Peter's age, enlargement of the prostate gland may cause an increased blood supply to that part of the bladder which is stretched over an enlarged prostate. This bleeds easily. Other causes of prostatic enlargement or disease, including infection or cancer of the prostate, may also cause bleeding. Stones in the urinary tract, whether in the kidney, pelvis, the ureter or the bladder, will usually cause bleeding and pain. The pain is colicky and may well be very severe.

Blood in the urine may also signal tumours in the bladder, kidney or prostate. Both the bladder and the kidney frequently grow benign tumours, but these always need careful investigation and, frequently, removal.

Bladder warts are particularly common, and although initially benign, may turn malignant if not treated. Cancerous growths may also occur in the bladder, kidney and the prostate.

Finally, a host of other unusual problems can cause blood in the urine, ranging from the potentially serious – including blood diseases that may cause problems with blood clotting – to the trivial, including small genital injuries or sores in either sex. If these bleed, the urine becomes contaminated with blood.

It turned out that Peter, like so many men in their fifties, had a benignly enlarged prostate. His even temperament ensured that he managed to keep smiling even through a series of uncomfortable examinations. At the end of these, he thanked everyone involved and said he was happy it wasn't anything more serious.

Look out for

joint pains

joint stiffness

swollen joints

tender joints

loss of weight

generalized feelings of ill health

muscle weakness

headache

pain and tenderness over the
forehead and temporal region

11
ACHES & PAINS
Arthritis

Osteoarthritis

James Titcombe, seventy, had worked on a farm from the time he was fifteen until he retired at sixty-five. He now hobbled across the road for a drink at the George and Dragon at lunchtime, returning in the evening at 6pm. His walking had become increasingly painful, but this didn't trouble him as much as the sleeplessness caused by his painful hips. Finally, he went to his doctor. 'I'm used to pain and stiffness in my knees and hips when I walk,' he said, 'but I can't take many more sleepless nights. I hope this isn't arthritis?'

When James was told that he was showing the classic signs of osteoarthritis, he gave a reply that would surprise most people. He said he was glad it 'wasn't arthritis'. To many people, arthritis means only rheumatoid arthritis. In fact, the word 'arthritis' simply means an inflamed joint: not a complete diagnosis, but the description of a symptom which has many different causes.

James had osteoarthritis, a degenerative disease in which the cartilage covering the surfaces of the bones is gradually worn away.

The more it erodes, the more the bones in the joint grind together. This loss of cushioning cartilage results in the pain and stiffness which follows the inflammation. Damage to the bone caused by osteoarthritis also stimulates the formation of cysts as well as small overgrowths of bone which make the pain worse. The pain starts by being worse in the morning, but as the day wears on, usually lessens. Later, it may be present the whole time, and an association with exercise may become obvious. The pain isn't consistent, but varies over the weeks or months.

Osteoarthritis tends to affect the spine, knees and hips in men, and the hands and fingers of women, but all joints in either sex may be affected. Contributory factors are family history, age, and excessive wear and tear (particularly in the damp and cold). Previous injury to a limb may encourage it, as may excessive weight. Obesity more often leads to arthritis of the knees than of the hips.

Rheumatoid arthritis

Marjorie Dean is a doctor's widow of fifty-five. When her husband first became ill, she began to feel unwell herself. If asked, she would say that she felt as if she had flu. She had all the tiredness, aches and pains of flu, but without the cough and snuffly nose. The symptoms lasted for weeks. Her appetite had disappeared and she was losing weight. She then noticed that several of her joints, usually the same joint on both sides of her body, were becoming painful and stiff, particularly in the morning. The joints were swollen and tender, but after a few weeks to describe them as being tender didn't do justice to the intense pain she felt when they were touched. Marjorie, remembering what she had learned from her husband's patients' illnesses, asked her doctor, 'Could this be rheumatoid?'

Yes. This is the classic start of rheumatoid arthritis, but in other cases the disease may begin more suddenly, with the joint symptoms of tenderness and stiffness being prominent from the beginning. The inflammatory arthritis of rheumatoid arthritis attacks the synovial membranes: the tissues which line the joint cavities. The inflammation results from abnormal changes in the patient's immune system, but what triggers these changes is unknown.

What is known is that the disease often runs in families, and is two or three times more common in women than in men. The relationship of rheumatoid arthritis to stress is still being debated; it is now thought to be less significant than was hitherto believed. While osteoarthritis becomes progressively more common the greater the age of a person, conversely, rheumatoid arthritis, although it may start at any time of life, most frequently begins in people between the ages of twenty-five and fifty.

While osteoarthritis is a degenerative disease that attacks the joints but leaves the rest of the body almost completely unaffected, rheumatoid arthritis is a generalized disease. The extreme joint tenderness, pain and stiffness are only some of its many features which may affect every system in the body.

Early diagnosis is important. If rheumatoid arthritis is treated from the beginning, it may prevent the deformities and crippling changes to the joints that are now well-recognized. Because there are so many different causes of arthritis, any arthritic symptoms should be shown to a doctor so that their importance may be assessed.

Arthritis is not only a symptom in various joint diseases, but it can be an early symptom of other diseases not obviously connected to joint disease.

POLYMYALGIA RHEUMATICA

Sixty-five-year-old Angela Tindall worked as
the manager of a travel agency. She retired,
opted to take travel vouchers as her leaving
present, and settled down to enjoy herself. On
her third Caribbean cruise in five years, she
developed sudden pain in her neck and the
muscles of her chest and shoulders. The pain
and stiffness were much worse in the morning,
or even after she had been lying on the lounger
by the swimming pool for an hour or two. She
was no better once she returned home. In
addition, she was losing weight, felt very ill and
depressed, and was running a fever each night.
She thought she might have cancer. Heavy with
foreboding, she went to see her doctor. 'Do I
have cancer?' she asked, and braced herself for
the answer.

The doctor examined her, did a simple blood test
known as an ESR estimation, which measures
the rate at which blood cells settle when blood
is suspended in a fine tube, and asked her to
wait for an hour. When she came back into

the consulting room, he gave her a broad grin
and said that he had excellent news.

The monstrously high ESR, the pattern of
the arthritic pains (with the same joints of the
upper limb being affected on both sides of the
body), the wasting of the muscles of her
shoulder girdle and her loss of appetite and
weight did not suggest that she had either
cancer or rheumatoid arthritis. He was almost
one hundred percent certain that Angela had
polymyalgia rheumatica, which is much more
common than generally realized. It normally
attacks the over-sixties, is rare in people under
fifty, and affects women twice as often as men.

The doctor said that even before he sent her to
a specialist to confirm his diagnosis, he wanted
to give Angela one warning. One in five of
people with polymyalgia rheumatica also suffer
from a condition known as temporal arteritis.

Temporal arteritis is an inflammation in the
arteries of the forehead and temporal region
of the head. It is not confined to those who
have polymyalgia. It is always important to
diagnose temporal arteritis early, as it is one
of the most crucial diagnoses in medicine. In

twenty-five percent of those cases of temporal arteritis that are not treated immediately, patients suffer damage to the artery leading to the retina of the eye.

If this artery is severely damaged by the inflammation, it is obliterated and the patients lose their sight. The blindness can be very sudden and permanent. If treatment is given immediately, patients retain their sight and all is well.

Temporal arteritis is also associated with a severe headache, which is felt over the area supplied by the inflamed arteries, and with an extreme tenderness over the scalp. The tenderness is often noticed when the hair is brushed or combed – simple tasks that suddenly become agonizing. Sometimes there is pain and tenderness over the face and jaw.

Treatment for both polymyalgia rheumatica and temporal arteritis is with steroids. The response is dramatic, but lower doses of these drugs may have to be continued for many months, or even a year or two.

LOOK OUT FOR

Headaches that Signal Other Problems

pain accompanied by
other symptoms, such as

fever • dizziness • nausea

vomiting • loss of appetite

change in vision

joint pains • muscle weakness

any change in mood or character

any loss of consciousness

is the headache present on waking?

is it persistent throughout the day?

does it vary in intensity?

is it getting worse?

was it of sudden onset?

is the scalp tender?

12
HEAD TROUBLE
Fainting and Headaches

DIZZINESS

Karen Wagstaff had a full figure and a ready smile but her eyes betrayed her anxiety. She went to see her doctor to ask him about another symptom doctors dread. 'I'm having dizzy turns,' she said, 'and I feel sick. What is it?'

Patients describe a wide variety of sensations as dizzy turns, ranging from true vertigo, when the world seems to be spinning round, to a simple feeling of lightheadedness. The latter includes a sensation of unsteadiness and a feeling of unreality; it may be very vague.

These symptoms may be caused by such conditions as anaemia, low blood pressure, obstruction to the blood supply to the head and neck, or anxiety (standing on a high ledge or tower can induce it). They may also be associated with palpitations or a sensation of an approaching faint coupled with the feeling that the world is turning black. Other patients may even label an unsteady and staggering gait or clumsiness as dizziness.

Karen's vertigo was of the spinning variety.

It had come on suddenly and was worse when she moved her head, but to her great relief, the giddiness and nausea were relieved by lying down. There was no pain, and no ringing in the ears (tinnitus). The doctor carried out a full neurological examination. He noted a flicker in the eyes but no other neurological symptoms. He diagnosed labyrinthitis, a viral complaint. After taking a few pills similar to seasickness tablets, Karen was as right as rain within three or four days.

Similar symptoms to Karen's, but of slower onset and associated with ringing in the ears and deafness, are classic signs of Menières Syndrome, a chronic condition of unknown cause. Vertigo may also result from damage to, or disease in, the central nervous system, whether the brain or spinal cord. Although the cause of Karen's trouble was easily diagnosed, dizziness often requires complex tests and a specialized examination.

Fainting

William Dean is a solitary fifty-five-year-old. He decided to attend his vicar's annual drinks party after a rushed day in the office, but hadn't eaten either lunch or tea. William was standing awkwardly, chatting to his fellow parishioners, when he started to feel hot and sweaty. The world became dark. The next thing he knew, he was lying on the floor while anxious people undid his collar, tie, and the waistband of his trousers. The next day he went to see the doctor. 'Everyone says I fainted,' he said, 'but how do I know I didn't have a stroke or heart attack?'

The doctor examined William carefully, took his blood pressure, which was a bit low, carried out an ECG (heart-tracing test), and arranged for full biochemical and blood tests. When William came back in a week's time, he was told all his results had been excellent. The only unusual abnormality was a low blood pressure.

His heart tracing was normal, and there was no evidence of any heart disease. He didn't have diabetes, and he wasn't anaemic. In addition, from looking at the back of William's eye, there was no evidence that he was likely to suffer from the type of arterial disease which might lead to a stroke. His cholesterol levels were excellent, and there was nothing to suggest that he was likely to suffer from early ageing of his arteries.

People are most likely to faint when they stand for a long time in the same place – particularly if they're hot, tired and haven't eaten recently. William had been tired and a bit anxious, hadn't eaten all day, and hadn't moved around much in the vicar's overheated room. All these factors, together with his permanently low blood pressure, favoured diagnosis of a simple faint. If William had any more trouble, however, he was told to go back to the doctor immediately.

Faints must be differentiated from seizures and heart disease, particularly when they result in a low pulse rate. The effect of a stroke does not wear off quickly, unlike those of the 'mini-stroke' known as a TIA (see page 184).

Headaches

Headaches are always worrying to patients. However, only rarely in the absence of other major symptoms do they indicate serious disease. Margaret Ransome, a fifty-five-year-old charity worker, had recently been suffering from headaches. These had come on after a cough and cold which hadn't entirely lifted. She had also complained of some nausea, so a neighbour suggested that she visit the doctor. The neighbour had heard that the combination of nausea and headaches sometimes indicated the presence of a brain tumour. Margaret went to see her doctor and said, 'I would be worried enough by any headache which lasted for a week or two, but I am particularly worried about this one as I am feeling sick the whole time. Do you think I have a brain tumour?'

The doctor listened to Margaret's story carefully, then examined her meticulously. He looked at the back of her eyes as well as checking her nervous system. He said she had done just the right thing by coming to see him, but as with most patients who fear brain tumours, the explanation of the headache was much less sinister.

The clue to Margaret's headache was her infection – she had sinusitis. The nausea was the result of a post-nasal drip: a discharge from the back of the nose trickling down the throat. The doctor arranged a CAT scan of the sinuses (X-rays are not always helpful), which confirmed his diagnosis. After antibiotics, the trouble cleared up.

Tension headaches are the other common cause of an otherwise inexplicable but long-standing headache. These headaches tend to be felt right around the head, prompting patients to say, 'Doctor, I feel as if I have a tight band around my head.' In other cases, the headache spreads from the back of the head to behind the forehead. Usually, tension headaches, which are related to stress and worries, vary in intensity. There are periods when there is no pain. Headaches also complicate any infection that causes a fever. When a patient has a raised temperature, the headache is persistent and dull.

So far as it is possible to generalize, the

headache that results from a brain tumour gradually worsens and is most marked early in the morning, after the patient has been lying flat all night. As time passes, the headache is not only more painful, but it lasts longer, eventually all day.

A person with increased pressure in the head from a growing cancer may not only have a headache but may often feel nauseous and may vomit. Members of the patient's family are likely to notice a change in mood. There may be other incidental symptoms, including increased sleepiness, dizziness, an unsteady walk, blurred vision, slurred speech, forgotten words, neurological signs such as muscle weakness or changes in skin sensation, and sometimes seizures (convulsions or fits), which are the first sign of trouble.

The headaches of a stroke depend on the type of stroke sustained. The most dramatic stroke headaches are known as subarachnoid haemorrhage. These are of amazingly sudden onset – so sudden that patients who have suffered this type of stroke, in which the irritant blood seeps into the fluid bathing the brain (the cerebrospinal fluid, or CSF), say that they feel as if they have been hit suddenly across the head or neck. Headaches of very sudden onset should never be neglected.

There are plenty of other causes of headache, including those of migraine – a complete study in itself; cluster headaches; and headaches stemming from arthritic necks, diseased ears and rotten teeth.

Among the more dangerous infections in which headaches are an important symptom are meningitis (see page 188) and malaria.

STROKES

Dr Charles Finsberg is eighty-four. A brilliant scientist, he lived life to the full. Six years ago, he noticed a weakness in his left leg. He went to his doctor, who didn't think the condition ominous, but soon the weakness became more pronounced and also extended to his left arm. Dr Finsberg had been taking warfarin, an anticoagulant, following a recent hip replacement. Five years later, Dr Finsberg still takes an interest in the world but can no longer work. 'Doctor,' he asked, 'how long will I last?'

No one can predict how long Dr Finsberg will last, but as his stroke was an adverse effect of taking warfarin, his arteries may be in reasonable condition and he could well live longer than would otherwise have been the case.

A stroke follows the cutting off of the blood supply to a portion of the brain. The supply may be disrupted either by a thromboembolus (a clot) blocking a cerebral blood vessel, or by a haemorrhage (bleeding) from a ruptured vessel. In over eighty percent of cases, the stroke is ischaemic: it follows the formation of a clot. In Dr Finsberg's case, it was from a bleed presumably related to his warfarin.

Each year, over 100,000 people in England and Wales have strokes and about 60,000 deaths annually are the result of one. At any time, 300,000 people in the UK are disabled from a past stroke.

Dr Finsberg's weakness and the pattern of its development are common. Sometimes the muscular weakness may be very slight, no more than a sagging face, but the rule is that the more minor the stroke, the more urgently it needs treatment. Patients with minor strokes may be the easiest ones to help by way of preventing another stroke or disability.

As well as paralysis or weakness affecting one side of the body, one side of the face may sag. Patients may find it hard to find words, the voice may slur and there may be tingling in the affected limb. They may also be disorientated, confused and unable to recall where they are.

Any neurological symptom needs urgent investigation. One type of stroke, called a subarachnoid haemorrhage, is characterized by a sudden headache – like being hit over the head (see page 181). There would be fewer strokes if everyone over forty had regular blood pressure checks, and if they had a raised blood pressure, had it treated adequately. Whatever the patient's age group, weight should kept down and half an hour's exercise taken daily.

The effect of a stroke does not wear off quickly, unlike those of the 'mini-stroke' known as a transient ischaemic attack (TIA), in which a small clot temporarily blocks an artery in the brain. A TIA causes stroke-like symptoms that persist for a short time (a few hours at most) before disappearing completely. People who have TIAs should regard them as an ominous warning and take aspirin and/or Plavix to prevent a recurrence that could cause permanent damage.

Sudden blindness

While travelling to London on a hot day, Christine Ronald read *The Times* to while away the hours. The print became difficult to see as a shower of floaters (specks apparently drifting in front of her right eye) were joined by bright, flashing lights, like fireworks. Before she reached London, she had almost entirely lost the vision in her right eye. The flashing lights had given way to a dark curtain that cloaked her line of vision. Already so short-sighted that she needed pebble-thick spectacles, Christine inched her way first to the taxi rank, and from there went straight to the emergency department at Moorfields Eye Hospital. 'Why have I gone blind?' she asked.

Christine was suffering from a detached retina. The retina is the light-sensitive area at the back of the eye that receives images transmitted to the brain via the optic nerve. A tear in the retina may allow fluid from the cavity within the eyeball to ooze under it, separating it from the back of the eye. This disaster is more common in the very short-sighted, particularly if they have had a blow to the head. Some anecdotal evidence suggests that very hot weather and dehydration may also increase its likelihood.

Christine was treated with laser therapy and regained much of her sight. Retinal detachment is an emergency, so the earlier the treatment, the better the results. The symptoms – increase in floaters, a shower of flashing lights, a curtain coming down across the eye – need immediate expert attention. A detached retina is painless.

Sudden blindness can have many causes. Blockage of the central retinal artery, usually from an embolus (clot), causes a painless and immediate blindness in one eye. The clot can sometimes be dislodged by massage of the eye with the eyelids closed. Drawing off fluid from the eye may also occasionally cause the embolus to move, thereby restoring vision.

Blocking of the central retinal vein may occur in patients with diseases such as hypertension and diabetes. It has symptoms similar to occlusion of the retinal artery, but the blindness is not so sudden. The outlook is better than for those with blocked retinal arteries.

Amaurosis fugax is another cause of sudden blindness in one visual field (or part of one). Just as with retinal detachment, it seems as if a shutter has obscured vision for seconds or minutes (usually under five minutes). Very rarely, the symptoms may last up to twenty-four hours. There are many different causes for this, but the most common is a transient athero-thrombo-embolism, a TIA (see page 184), a clot in the artery that moves on. While this isn't the only cause of sudden transitory blindness, if diagnosed, it needs immediate treatment with aspirin, as do TIAs affecting other arteries.

A stroke may also cause sudden blindness, usually in both eyes, occasionally just in one. Acute glaucoma, associated with an increase in the pressure of the eye, may be a very painful cause of sudden vision loss. The eye is very inflamed, and emergency treatment is essential. Other causes include inflammation of the optic nerve, bleeding in the eyeball and temporal arteritis (see page 170). All are emergencies.

Meningococcal meningitis

If septicaemia is complicating meningitis, the patient may have a rash as well as the usual meningitis signs and symptoms. Meningitis must never be ruled out as a diagnosis because there is no rash; this can be, and sometimes is, a fatal mistake. The rash, when it starts, doesn't look like the standard picture of a meningococcal rash (*i.e.* a purple bruise), but starts as tiny dark-pink or red spots. Later they grow larger and develop a purple bruise-like appearance and colour.

In adults and older children, early meningitis symptoms may be mistaken for flu

- headache
- fever
- aches and pains
- neck stiffness: painful when the head is bowed and the chin placed on the chest
- dislike of light
- irritability and change in personality
- vomiting
- confusion
- fits

Symptoms in babies, and small children

- irritability
- change in child's response to parents
- difficult to rouse, lethargic
- fever
- diarrhoea, vomiting
- a high-pitched cry
- dislike of light

In small children and babies the hands and feet may be cold, despite the fever, and the skin pale and blotchy. In babies, the fontanelles, the soft areas in the baby's skull, may bulge.

- Never rule out meningitis because there is no rash

- Never wait for a rash to develop

- Remember, the rash of meningococcal meningitis doesn't fade when pressed beneath glass

LOOK OUT FOR

red palms • spider naevi

an obvious fine tremor • limb-wasting

with central weight gain • later – jaundice

genital atrophy and loss of secondary

sexual characteristics

in males loss of libido and potency

excessive, inexplicable tiredness

increasing indigestion

bloating • loss of appetite

abdominal pain • unreliable bowels

Don't Miss

liver failure is insidious – for fifteen years the liver
may be failing but the only outward signs may be
increased tiredness, a faint tremor, red palms and
spider naevi, but no significant generalized symptoms.

13
LIVER PROBLEMS

LIVER PROBLEMS IN MEN

Colin was a Celt. He was brilliant. When he was a boy at the local academy in his Scottish Highland town his brains were legendary, and an envy of all the other mothers. He won a scholarship to Edinburgh University, where he did well, but not as well as his parents had hoped. At the university, where he was studying medicine, he met others who were as clever as he was; his colleagues were equally charming and he no longer stood out as the star. Although he shone in group discussions, and his lecturers had picked him out as a winner, his exam results were, surprisingly, disappointing.

In Edinburgh he didn't only learn medicine, but he also understood why it was that his father found three or four glasses of whisky such a relief after a hard day at the distillery. From the very first drink or two he had had with his new mates at the university, he knew that alcohol was the key to relaxation. It was an unusual day when he didn't drink four or five pints and a glass of whisky or two.

After Edinburgh he started on the usual round

of junior hospital appointments, but bright as his clinical opinions were, and as happily as he achieved a rapport with his patients, his promotion wasn't as fast as it might have been. He never took his higher exams and his seniors were repeatedly rather disturbed about the stories they heard of his drinking bouts. They wondered whether they could account for the occasional black eye.

Colin disappeared into a small practice in Sutherland. His patients soon learnt that he gave a better opinion in the morning than after lunch, and that sometimes at night it might be as well to call the neighbouring doctor from ten miles away. However, Colin remained – or so it seemed – perfectly fit, but about twelve years after he started in practice he was beginning to find that he was tiring easily, and his long-suffering wife was complaining about his increasing girth, his prematurely aged face and his lack of enthusiasm for sex. Colin blamed his indigestion and his failing potency on tiredness and pre-occupations about his patients. 'Anyway,' he said, having had a couple of quick drinks, 'it doesn't really matter, we're both getting older.'

Colin was also developing the shakes. His eyes had become baggy, his face coarsened and he had noticed red veins on his abdomen, chest and face. The veins were unusual, like a spider. They had a red centre forming the body of a spider and wavy legs protruding from it. When the body was pressed by the end of a pencil, the legs paled. He was also beginning to suffer from a fine tremor. The tremor was like that of someone who is anxious. It wasn't the slow, coarse shake of someone with Parkinson's Disease.

By now, he didn't only have indigestion, but was feeling sick every morning. His wife, Morag, was able to hear him retching in the bathroom after he had shaved. He didn't eat breakfast nor enjoyed lunch. One day the indigestion he had had for years seemed to be worse; he vomited, but it wasn't only his last drink that came back, but pints of blood. Colin was flown in the air ambulance to Inverness where oesophageal varices were diagnosed. These are varicose veins in the gullet that frequently form as the result of cirrhosis of the liver obstructing the usual venous drainage.

There are several different types of people that

become alcoholics. Although Colin displayed many of the symptoms of alcoholism and the signs of liver failure, it is an unfair assumption to believe that everyone who has cirrhosis is also a heavy drinker. Cirrhosis of the liver is frequently the result of infection by hepatitis B or C virus. Recently, a surprising number of people who don't drink, and have never been infected by hepatitis B or C, have developed fatty liver disease that in time will progress to cirrhosis. They haven't drunk too much, but rather they have eaten too much. In all probability they carry the gene for the metabolic syndrome.

The metabolic syndrome has been observed for many years, but only recently has it been named and its importance understood. It is the result of abnormalities in the effect that insulin has on every cell in the body. The obesity is frequently coupled with high blood pressure, a susceptibility to diabetes, high levels of cholesterol and triglycerides in the blood. Few people understand that the combination of increasing central obesity and the metabolic syndrome may result in genetically vulnerable people developing cirrhosis of the liver if they overeat, even if they don't drink a drop of alcohol. This problem is more common in women than in men such as Colin, who was a drinker.

Colin's personality was typical of one group of heavy drinkers who turn to alcohol for emotional support once they have to face up to the realities of life, or who feel socially insecure. His father was a heavy drinker and Colin took to whisky as a young duck takes to water. Colin was a clever, intellectual, goal-seeking person who set himself high standards and had revelled in the regard of friends and neighbours when he was young. He enjoyed the status of being a big fish in a small pond, and couldn't cope when he was a standard-sized fish in a lake. The greater world of university had exposed him to his equals, his confidence needed boosting, and alcohol was the easiest and most readily available crutch.

Characteristically, the cirrhosis came on slowly and insidiously. For many years he had no troubles at all but then he began to age prematurely and put on weight; his potency flagged and he developed a shake. He also began to vomit in the mornings. There are three main causes for early-morning vomiting: pregnancy — clearly not the cause in Colin's case — excessive anxiety — a possibility that might have contributed to Colin's problems — and alcoholism. Alcoholics develop gastritis as well as cirrhosis.

Colin was unlucky that the first serious symptom of his cirrhosis was a bleeding oesophageal varicose vein. As the liver shrinks and hardens, it interferes with the blood circulation in the area, and the back pressure in the veins around the oesophagus induces varicosities (varicose veins). Bleeding from these is a frequent cause of death as a result of liver failure.

Among other signs of liver failure are thickening of the palms (Dupuytren's contracure) that draws the fingers downwards so that the hands become claw-like. Liver failure also produces bright red palms, probably because the liver disease results in an increase in the amount of oestrogen circulating in the patient, whether they are male or female. Men suffer testicular and penile atrophy, and large breasts. The muscles in their limbs shrink and their tummies expand. They gradually lose their body hair.

Although there is little doubt about the cause of Colin's liver failure, it is a grave diagnostic error to assume that all cirrhosis is the result of alcoholism. Hepatitis C and B also cause liver failure and in both, as in alcohol-related liver failure, early symptoms are virtually non-existent. Nor is it right to assume that all heavy drinkers will develop cirrhosis or liver disease. Most heavy drinkers will develop some adverse side effects from alcohol, but only in about one in five or six will this lead to cirrhosis of the liver.

The amount that a man who is vulnerable to alcohol may drink before developing signs and symptoms of cirrhosis varies enormously. In men there is certainly a dose-related factor; the amount drunk, and for how long it has been drunk, do matter, but no hard or fast guidelines as to quantities of drink or years of drinking can be laid down.

In men the government limits of 28 units a week is a cautious one, but one that is likely to save men from developing cirrhosis, even if their livers are vulnerable to alcohol. The problem when setting a limit is that the social therapeutic dose that induces the click — the relaxed feeling brought about by a glass at the end of the day — is very close to the level at which regularly consumed alcohol becomes toxic.

Women's sensitive livers

Mary was a fragile, serious woman who had moved from her provincial university to a good job in a medical public relations agency. She soon adapted what she had learnt while taking her degree in bio-sciences to writing copy for the pharmaceutical companies. She had a pleasant, if quiet, social manner, was popular, even if not overtly gregarious. She made a good hostess when the latest drug needed to be introduced to a cynical press and well-informed doctors. Mary looked around at her colleagues in the agency and worried about the quantity they drank — not only when they went out clubbing on Fridays and Saturdays, but even during midweek meetings and after work every day. Mindful of the government's strictures on alcohol consumption, she kept her intake down to one or two units a day, and congratulated herself that she wasn't like many other women. She was always the sober one after a boozy lunch, and was the person delegated to drive everyone else home from a good dinner.

Mary married, had a child, but continued to work. By now she was important in the medical public relations world and was a partner in a medium-sized firm. She wondered why it was becoming more and more tiring to carry out her duties. She vaguely noticed that her appetite wasn't what it was and that her coffee cup rattled in its saucer as a result of a shake. Initially, she thought that it was because she was sleeping badly as she was worrying about her work. Her doctor was puzzled about her symptoms but wisely didn't accept any of the obvious explanations. When he ordered blood tests he cast the net wide and included liver function tests. Both he and Mary were astounded to find that she had evidence of advanced liver disease.

Whereas Colin's case was that of the typical male alcoholic from a heavy-drinking background and a stressed life, Mary's history could only have affected a woman suffering from alcoholic disease. In women, unlike in men, there is no such thing as a typical history that may lead to liver disease. Even a drink a day can be enough to occasionally bring it on in a pre-menopausal woman.

The music hall and stage female drunk is usually represented as a short, overweight, red-faced, blousy woman who props herself up against the bar and drinks until closing time. Often she is depicted as being tearful or aggressive, sometimes as being sexually predatory. Every text book will tell its readers that women can drink only half as much as men, since they have less of the necessary enzymes that metabolise alcohol. It is said that they become drunk more readily (they absorb alcohol faster than men) and sober up more slowly because of this lack of enzymes. Furthermore, their variable hormone levels result in their resistance to alcohol depending on the time of the month.

The other type of standard heavy drinking associated with women is that of the 'ladettes' who join the lads in the clubs and bars at the weekend. Even more than men, they drink before they go to the party to give them the necessary boost to their confidence and (since they have less testosterone) the drive to join an assembled company of total strangers in a night club. They drink such huge quantities that any older doctor would assume that if they had the propensity to develop cirrhosis they would be bound to do so. But in women, as in men, there must be a genetic vulnerability to alcohol before developing it after heavy drinking. Some women will develop evidence of liver disease earlier than men, hence the increasing numbers of young women being seen with cirrhosis in hospital outpatients departments.

There are two groups of women who may lapse into alcoholic liver disease while hardly noticing it or it being noticed by friends and relatives as it develops. Housewives, bored and lonely, may help themselves to an increasing but not obviously excessive number of glasses of wine or, if of an older generation, sherry, before meals. They forget that even to a greater extent than in men everyone's tolerance to alcohol differs, and without ever being drunk or drunken they may develop liver disease.

Mary was an extreme example of the vulnerability of some women to alcohol. It may be genetic; it certainly can have a racial component. In some towns in which there is a large South Asian population an increasing number of modest-drinking younger women are attending gastrointestinal clinics with early liver disease. As Mary's case shows, this phenomenon isn't related to any one race or any one drinking pattern.

Some women are like Mary and may develop liver disease although they drink no more than one unit a day. It is rare but worrying. The only consolation is that if women remain exceptionally sober when young, they will be able to drink more freely once they reach the menopause and their tolerance to alcohol increases.

Whether male or female, whether a potential Colin or Mary, or merely the man or woman in the street, there are some people who may not develop liver disease if they drink, but will feel most unwell, even after a glass or two. This is a genetic characteristic that runs in some families. It is akin to the characteristic of some Far Eastern races that don't have the enzymes to metabolise alcohol easily, so that they readily become flushed and sweaty after the first drink or two.

Other people with a very low alcohol

tolerance suffer from ALDH polymorphism. This is also an enzyme deficiency. After a drink, sometimes before even the second drink, they feel unwell, possibly irritable and aggressive, and have a bad hangover. Many of these patients have Jewish genes. In those of pure Jewish stock as many as one in four may carry this gene. Cynics say that this is why the approach to drinking alcohol in Jewish people has varied down the ages, and cite the fact that wine figured prominently in the new testaments, but is now decried by some Orthodox sects. Experience has taught Jewish people that a great many are going to feel very unwell after very little alcohol.

Look out for

For Deafness
complaints that others mumble and no longer speak clearly • grumbles that actors on the stage or screen are no longer taught diction • the radio isn't loud enough • parties are hell – you can't hear a word anyone says • pleas for old-fashioned, quiet restaurants – now no one can have a proper conversation

For Fading Taste and Smell (Intimately Linked Senses)
an inability to smell gas • failing interest in gourmet food and increasing desire to eat nursery food • increasing reliance on spoonfuls of mustard, lashings of salt and a love of spices • muttering about nothing tasting the way it used to • derogatory comments about supermarket food compared with fresh garden vegetables • a decreasing interest in wine and increasing interest in spirits

For Failing Sight
vision failing faster in one eye than the other • inability to read number plates at thirty-five yards • an increasing need to have stronger lights • loss of peripheral vision that may denote glaucoma • loss of central vision that can be a sign of macular degeneration • fuzziness of vision, difficulty in recognition, a halo around objects, easy dazzling – these may be signs of cataracts

14

FADING SENSES
IN OLDER PEOPLE
Loss of Taste, Smell,
Deafness and Failing Sight

LOSS OF SMELL, TASTE AND HEARING

George Harrison couldn't have been a more typical wine merchant. Immaculately dressed, well educated and well travelled, he was as much at home at wine tastings as he was in the smartest London clubs. The firm of wine merchants founded by him prospered. When retirement beckoned he sold it to a conglomerate for an immense sum of money. He no longer had to be concerned about the mortgage on his London flat or the debts owed by his farm in the country, but he did have worries. One day he went to see his doctor about his loss of hearing, and also mentioned that he hadn't been able to smell adequately for five or six years.

The loss of smell is the first of the senses to fade in old age. Technically known as hypogeusia, it may be associated with damage to a cranial nerve or a centre in the brain as a result of disease, including the degenerative diseases of age, stroke or an injury. The ability to taste is closely related to that of smell. People think that they have a very good palate, but in fact they have a perfectly normal palate in that they are usually able to taste all the basic flavours such as salt, sweetness, sourness and bitterness.

The subtlety of tastes, the difference between lamb and beef, claret and burgundy, or even white merlot and a blousy chardonnay is an aspect of smell rather than taste. The investigations showed that George's taste, the ability of his mouth to notice the difference between sweet and sour, was unaltered. They also showed that he had no palate in the wine merchant's use of the word at all. George could no longer tell sherry from port or mosel from claret. How did he manage? He admitted that for years he had been going around wine tastings, picking the brains of those who had tasted the wine before him. He then cheated by filling in his assessment forms according to the gossip in the room. He even smiled when the doctor told him that there was nothing that could be done for his taste and smell. George was rich and was reassured by the knowledge that only he and his doctor knew that he could no longer taste the wine he sold.

The story of George's hearing was equally

unusual. Although hearing is the last sense to leave someone as they lapse into unconsciousness before dying, and they frequently continue to hear conversation even after they appear to be unconscious, it is an almost inevitable part of ageing.

There is one form of deafness that among all the mammals is suffered only by humans. About one in ten people when older develop otosclerosis. This alters the nature of the links in the small chain of bones that transmit the vibrations from the eardrum, so that the impulses they stimulate in the nerves can no longer be transmitted to the brain. Otosclerosis is one of the few forms of deafness in the elderly that can be corrected by surgery.

George was one of the one in ten old people whose deafness could be helped by surgery. He had an operation on his ears. Once his otosclerosis had been dealt with, he was able to hear more clearly the opinions of his friends and rivals about the wine he was judging and buying, even though he still couldn't taste it.

FAILING SIGHT

Marion Gibson was an artist. Every year she held an exhibition that attracted the best-known art critics who gave Marion's annual work a detailed and laudatory write-up. Gradually her work no longer displayed its sense of colour, brightness and originality and the reviews became shorter and more perfunctory. The critics still attended the exhibitions because they met their friends and it was a good party, but the press coverage afterwards was limited. One year they went along as usual, expecting to drink champagne and to be polite, but they were astounded that all the old vigour and vitality had returned to Marion's paintings. Her reviews were ecstatic. Only her doctors knew the answer.

When Marion visited an ophthalmologist he immediately detected the cataracts that had changed her vision. He arranged for her to have them dealt with and promised her that soon she would again be seeing as well as she did when an eighteen-year-old. The ophthalmologist assured Marion that there was not any longer any nonsense about allowing the cataracts to ripen, or of prescribing pebble spectacles after surgery to remove a cataract. The doctor reassured her that pebble spectacles were instruments from a forgotten age. Now a neatly folded lens could be slipped into each of her eyes and her vision would be restored.

One afternoon Marion answered the call of the ophthalmologist and visited a nearby hospital. She was given a local anaesthetic, and the ophthalmologist made such a small incision in her eye that not even a stitch was later needed to repair it. The hardened lens was pulverised and sucked out and immediately a new Perspex lens was slipped in its place. When the pads were removed from Marion's eyes, she could focus perfectly, although she noticed initially that everything was tinted blue. Marion had an hour or two's rest during which time her usual sense of colour was restored. She discovered her vision was better than it had been for forty years. She could even read a book without spectacles and tell the time from the distant church clock.

There are now modern implantable lenses that

are able to cope with both distant and near vision. Marion's paintings at her next exhibition astounded the critics. Her old sense of colour had returned.

If the sense of smell and taste is the first victim of ageing, and hearing is the last to go entirely, loss of visual acuity is almost inevitable once people reach their seventies. In some cases this is related to macular degeneration, the wearing out of the retina that is akin to the wearing out of a well-used suit or an old pair of pyjamas. Although research on macular degeneration is proceeding apace, until recently not much could be done to produce any lasting improvement.

There are two types of age-related macular degeneration — wet and dry. Wet macular degeneration is the result of new blood vessels growing in the choroid's rich vascular bed and leaking. The bleeding separates the layers of the eyes so that vision becomes increasingly obscured. The dry type is just progressive disintegration of the layers of the retina. The wet type has always been the more dreaded variety as it develops more quickly. It accounts for only ten per cent of cases. Recently, two treatments for it have been introduced. One may delay its progress in a minority of cases, but only for months rather than years. In 2006 an injection of a drug into the eye every month has been found to inhibit the development of wet macular degeneration. The problem is that the expense is heavy, and the inconvenience to the patient considerable. The dry type of age-related macular degeneration accounts for ninety per cent of cases. The good news is that the reduction in vision usually never reaches the stage where all sight is lost, although it is severely restricted. The bad news is that as yet there is no treatment at all.

Fortunately, only a minority of people suffer enough macular degeneration for it to destroy their sight, but many others are inconvenienced by it. However, almost invariably everyone over seventy has some degree of cataract, as Marion had. It creeps on insidiously. Slowly the ageing person accepts that they need a stronger light to read, are dazzled by oncoming car headlights, and can no longer adjust their vision so rapidly when changing from looking at someone at a distance to admiring the person they are chatting to across the table.

One of the stranger features of a cataract is that it alters colour perception. The world becomes greyer, and the pictures by an artist with cataracts are less vibrant. This had happened to Marion. In Biblical and Shakespearean times loss of vision was accepted as part of growing older. Sir Harold Ridley, a British surgeon, devised the implanted lens. It has changed old age for over two hundred million people worldwide since Ridley introduced it. Now, at last, there is good news for sufferers from one sort of macular degeneration. Expensive, but once the boundaries of medicine begin to be pushed back, the process becomes faster and faster, and the cost less and less.

INDEX

ALSO BY DR TOM STUTTAFORD

TAKING IT EASY

Relax, put your feet up and take a short time out of your stress-ridden life to read this book. Here, *Times* columnist Dr Tom Stuttaford, one of our leading medical writers, brings together his knowledge and experience of life to explore the universal issue of stress. He explains its physical and psychological signs and symptoms, as well as the diseases it causes, revealing the way in which it erodes the quality of our lives.

Divorce, death, sex, marriage, moving house and even house repairs are key factors in generating stress. As well as exploring the consequences of trying to fit too much in without taking enough time out, Stuttaford analyzes the psychology of common events and situations and how they can affect the tension we feel. Armed with a more in-depth understanding of how to negotiate life's rollercoasters, footloose and fancy free, you can look forward to better health and happiness.

ISBN 978 1 904435 67 9
Price £6.99

Copies of *Taking It Easy* are available from all good bookshops or can be ordered direct from the publishers on credit card hotline number 01933 443862.